Everybody's Guide to Cosmetic Plastic Surgery

Lachlan Currie

Disclaimer

This publication is intended as a self-help publication. The information contained in this publication is not medical advice for any individual and does not substitute for a medical opinion from a registered practitioner. All the information within this publication is the express opinion of the author based on his experience and research. The accuracy of the information cannot be guaranteed, though every effort has been made to ensure it is an accurate reflection of current concepts in cosmetic plastic surgery. The conditions, operations and complications described are not exhaustive and many important considerations may have been omitted in order to keep the text concise. None of the information is intended to be used to treat or diagnose illness, merely to encourage individuals to seek accredited medical advice from a medical professional. The author is not responsible for any injury, illness or death resulting from the utilization of the treatments, procedures or products discussed in this publication.

Copyright © 2007. Lachlan Currie. All rights reserved.

Copyright notice: No part of this publication may be reproduced in any form, by photocopy, microfilm, xerography, or any other means which are now known or yet to be invented, or incorporated into any information retrieval system, electronic or mechanical, without the written permission of the copyright owner.

First Published 2007

Gladiator Publishing

ISBN: 978-0-9556809-0-8

Contents

Foreword — 9

1. Botox. — 11

The History of botox	12
Who benefits from botox?	14
How does botox work?	15
Facial Aesthetics	15
Medical uses for botox	16
Contra-indications to botox	16
What does botox injection involve?	16
What are the risks of botox?	17
Botox injection sites	18
Botox summary	19

2. Fillers. — 20

The history of fillers	20
The uses of fillers	22
Types of filler	23
Temporary fillers	24
Collagen fillers	24
Hyaluronic acid fillers	27
Fat as a filler	29
Permanent/ semi-permanent fillers	30

Injection techniques	32
Facial regions treated with fillers	34
Glabella lines	34
Forehead lines	35
Crow's feet and eyes	36
Nasolabial fold	36
Lips and marionette lines	37
Contraindications to fillers	39
Adverse effects of fillers	39
Fillers summary	41

3. Facial Peels. 42

Who benefits from a facial peel?	42
What does a facial peel involve?	42
What are the risks of facial peels?	44
Facial peels summary	47

4. Laser. 48

The cosmetic uses of laser	48
Laser skin resurfacing	**49**
How does laser skin resurfacing work?	49
What does laser skin resurfacing involve?	50
What are the risks of laser treatment?	51
Laser skin resurfacing summary	53
Laser Hair Removal	**54**

Contents

How does laser hair removal work?	54
What does laser hair removal involve?	56
Laser hair removal summary	57

5. Facelift. — 58

What does a facelift involve?	59
Types of facelift	64
What are the risks of a facelift?	66
Facelift summary	69

6. Brow Lift. — 70

Who benefits from a browlift?	70
What is a browlift?	71
What does an endoscopic brow lift involve?	76
What are the risks involved with brow lift surgery?	77
Brow lift summary	79

7. Eyelid Surgery – Blepharoplasty. — 80

Who benefits from eyelid surgery?	80
What does eyelid surgery aim to do?	81
What does eyelid surgery involve?	83
What are the risks involved with eyelid sugery?	84
Eyelid surgery summary	87

8. Nose Surgery – Rhinoplasty. — 88

Who benefits from nose surgery?	88
How is a rhinoplasty done?	91
What does nasal surgery involve for the patient?	95
What are the risks of nasal surgery?	96
Rhinoplasty summary	98

9. Prominent Ear Correction – Otoplasty — 99

How are prominent ears corrected	100
What does the ear surgery involve	103
What are the risks of ear surgery	104
Otoplasty summary	106

10. Breast Reduction Surgery — 107

Who benefits from a breast reduction?	107
How is a breast reduction done?	108
Vertical scar technique	108
Inverted T scar technique	111
What does a breast reduction involve?	115
What are the risks of breast reduction surgery?	116
Breast reduction summary	120

11. Breast Lift Surgery – Mastopexy. — 121

Who benefits from a breast lift?	121
What does breast lift surgery involve?	124
What does a breast lift involve for the patient?	129

What are the risks of having a breast lift?	130
Breast lift surgery summary	132

12. Breast Augmentation Surgery. — 133

Who benefits from breast augmentation surgery?	133
Types of breast implant?	134
Implant shape	135
Implant shell	136
Implant size	137
The silicone debate	138
Implants and breast cancer	140
Incisions for breast implants	141
What does breast augmentation involve?	145
What are the risks of augmentation surgery?	145
Breast augmentation summary	149

13. 'Tummy tuck' – Abdominoplasty. — 151

Who benefits from a tummy tuck?	151
How is an abdominoplasty done?	153
What does an abdominoplasty involve?	159
What are the risks of an abdominoplasty?	160
Abdominoplasty summary	162

14. Liposuction. — 163

Who benefits from liposuction?	163

How is liposuction done? 164

What does liposuction involve for the patient? 165

What are the risks of liposuction? 166

Liposuction summary 168

15. Choosing a cosmetic surgeon 169

16. Glossary 173

Cosmetic and Plastic Surgery

Cosmetic surgery is performed to reshape *normal* structures of the body in order to improve the patient's appearance. Reconstructive plastic surgery is performed on *abnormal* structures of the body. It is generally performed to improve function, but may also be done to create a normal appearance. Cosmetic surgery refers to any surgery that is designed to improve a patient's cosmetic appearance.

The word "plastic" is derived from the Greek word *plastikos* meaning to mold or to shape. It literally means surgery to mould or shape the body. It has nothing to do with plastic polymers or their use, which share the same Greek derivative.

Many people wish to improve their appearance. Modern cosmetic surgery has evolved into a specialist field which involves the use of numerous reliable techniques that allow safe improvements to be made to the face and body. This book outlines procedures commonly used by cosmetic and plastic surgeons. It also explains the risks and benefits of each procedure so that individuals can make balanced, informed decisions before embarking on complex surgery.

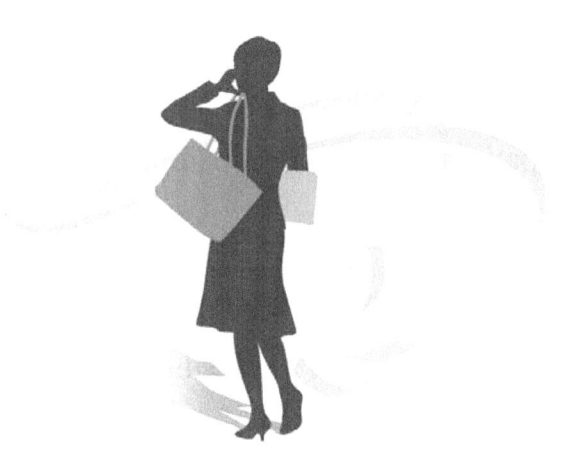

1. Botox®

The History of Botox®

Botulinum toxin is one of the most poisonous naturally occurring substances in the world, and it is the most toxic protein known to man. It is a neurotoxin produced by the bacterium *Clostridium botulinum*. The name botulism comes from the Latin word "botulus" meaning "sausage". The term was first used by a German physician, Muller, in 1870 to describe the bacterium which caused poisoning by growing in badly handled or prepared meat products. Edward Schantz cultured *Clostridium botulinum* bacteria in 1944 and isolated the toxin in 1949. The toxin was first used to treat eye muscle disorders in 1980 and then for facial spasm in 1989. It was noticed that facial lines and wrinkles were reduced in these patients.

In April 2002 the FDA announced the approval of botulinum toxin type A to be used to improve the appearance of moderate-to-severe frown lines between the eyebrows (glabellar lines). In 2006 there were 4.1 million cosmetic Botox® procedures carried out in America. It is now the most popular cosmetic surgery procedure performed.

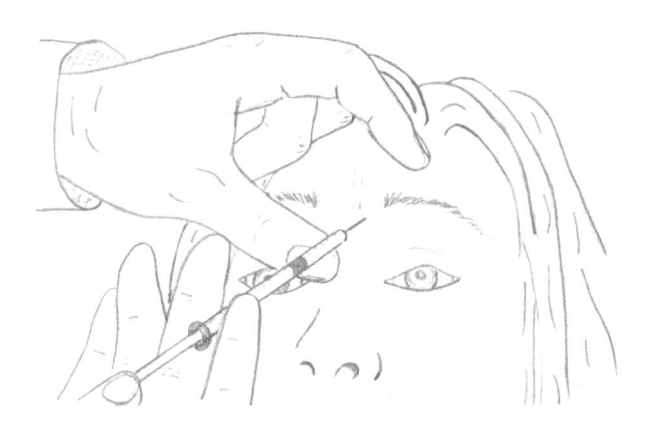

Although botulinum toxin is possibly the most toxic substance known, poisoning is rare. The lethal dose for an adult is about 70 nanograms. A few hundred grams (the content of a soft drink can) could theoretically kill every human on earth. Food-borne botulism usually results from ingestion of food that has become contaminated with spores in an oxygen free environment (such as a tin can), allowing the spores to germinate and grow into bacteria. The bacteria produce toxin. It is the ingestion of the toxin that causes botulism, not ingestion of the spores or the organism. One in five patients with botulism die. Death is generally secondary to respiratory failure due to paralysis of the respiratory muscles, so treatment consists of antitoxin administration and artificial ventilation.

Injection of Botox® is safe due to the extreme dilution of the toxin used. A patient would have to be injected with the contents of at least 30 vials to reach a toxic dose. A vial of Botox® costs about £130 in the UK , so this error is highly unlikely.

Interestingly Botulin toxin has always been considered an inferior agent for chemical warfare since it degrades rapidly on exposure to air, and therefore an attacked with the toxic aerosol would be useless. It is not therefore a potential terrorist threat. It is reported that in 1961 the CIA saturated some of Fidel Castro's favorite brand of cigars with botulinum toxin for a possible assassination attempt (Operation Mongoose). The cigars were never used, but when tested years later were found to still be effective.

Who benefits from Botox®?

Botox® injections can improve fine lines and wrinkles. Botox® works best in people who develop facial wrinkles when they smile or laugh. The injections will have less effect on deep facial lines which are present at all times. The best candidates for Botox® are younger patients whose skin is still relatively elastic. It may help delay the onset of skin wrinkling. Older patients will get some improvement, but may not get complete resolution of deeper facial lines. The effects of Botox® injections last for only three or four months, but the treatments can be repeated. Forehead lines and "crow's feet" around the eyes are the most commonly treated areas.

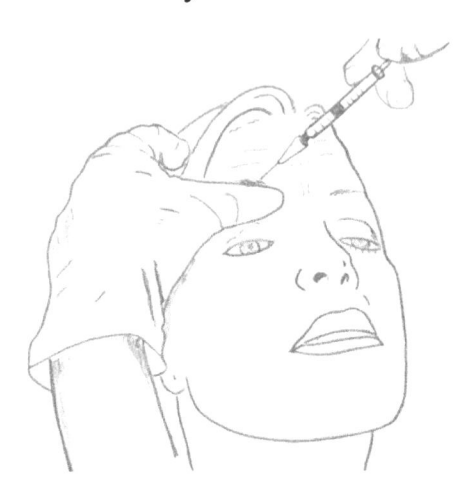

How does Botox® work?

Botox® injections contain botulinum toxin. This is a protein produced by the bacteria. It blocks the release of acetylcholine, which normally transmits messages from the nerves to the muscles to make them contract and move. Once transmission has been blocked, muscles relax. The effect is completely reversible and generally lasts for a few months in most clinical uses. The degree of relaxation in a given muscle depends on the dose injected into each area. Wrinkles in the skin are produced by muscles below the skin contracting. The wrinkles become permanent over time, like a book spine which is folded too many times and is left with a permanent mark. Paralysing the facial muscles with Botox® prevents this folding process and skin wrinkles will improve.

Facial Aesthetics

Botox® will eradicate wrinkles. It also allows an expert to reshape facial features by relaxing some muscles whilst leaving others functional. If placed below the eyebrow the muscular relaxation will raise the position of the eyebrow. The arch of the eyebrow can be shaped by using graduated doses across the forehead. Botox® can also be used to eliminate unwanted facial expressions, such as a snarl. It also improves the appearance of muscular bands in the neck (platysmal bands).

Medical Uses For Botox®

Botox® has been used to treat a variety of medical problems. These include excessive sweating, drooling, and muscle spasm after strokes.

Contra-indications To Botox®

Botox® should be avoided in patients with peripheral neuromuscular disease, patients on amininoglycoside antibiotics, patients with inflammatory skin conditions, during pregnancy and in lactating mothers.

What does Botox® injection involve?

The surgeon will inject the areas of the face that have wrinkles. The injection is similar to a sharp pin prick. The Botox® takes a couple of days to have effect and the facial lines and wrinkles will become progressively less noticeable. The injection site will usually not be perceptible by the next day. The effects start to fade away after about three months.

What are the risks of Botox®?

Local complications such as swelling and bruising can occur, but they usually resolve within a week. If too much Botox® is used in a large area, patients can be left with slightly expressionless faces, with very little emotional content. Proficient practitioners will try to avoid this. If Botox® is placed in the wrong areas, it can also have some undesirable effects. For example it can cause the eyebrows to drop excessively, or the eyelid to droop. If used around the mouth, it can sometimes cause a slightly asymmetric smile.

The Botox® product information sheet states that it contains Human Serum Albumin (HSA) and advises that there is a theoretical risk of viral and prion (which cause Creutzfeldt-Jakob disease) transmission. No such cases have ever been reported.

Botox Injection Sites

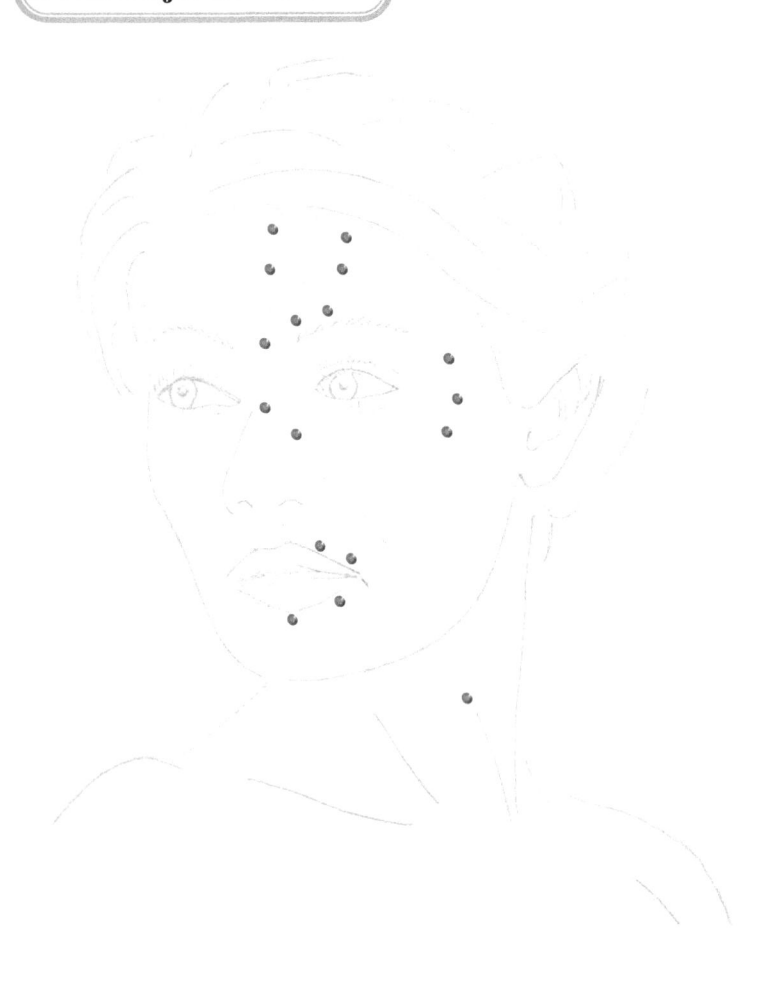

BOTOX® INJECTIONS	
Cost	UK: £ 200 - £400 US: $200 - $400
Anaesthetic	nil or topical cream
Hospital stay	nil
Recovery	1 day
Risks	Bruising (transient) Eyelid droop (temporary) Eyebrow drop (temporary) Facial asymmetry (temporary)

2. Fillers

The History of Fillers

In 2005 over one million people used temporary fillers for facial rejuvenation, and this number is increasing every year. It is the third most popular cosmetic surgery procedure in the United States after Botox injection and laser hair removal.

Fat was probably the first filler to be used over 100 years ago. Fat injection reportedly started in 1893 when a German physician Franz Neuber used a small piece of upper arm fat to build up the face of a patient whose cheek had a large pit caused by tuberculosis. Paraffin and silicone were used at the turn of the 19th century, but these lost popularity with the realisation that they could produce granulomas (small nodules) when injected directly into the tissue. These early products were banned by the FDA. In the 1970's collagen was approved for use as a filler. Collagen is a protein found in most human tissues and forms a substantial part of the normal skin structure. The early products were manufactured from bovine (cow) collagen. These products have been used extensively but there is a risk of allergy to the non-human material when it is injected. More recently human-derived collagen products, manufactured from donor skin, have been approved for use.

Hyaluronic acid was first approved for use as a filler in 2003. Hyaluronic acid is also found naturally in the skin. It provides structure to the dermis around the collagen fibres and maintains moisture within the skin. The earliest products were non-animal derived. The hyaluronic acid was produced by bacteria and then cross-linked in the manufacturing process to produce a gel which can be injected into tissue. It lasts for several months before being broken down by the body's normal degradation systems, and there is little risk of allergy. There is now a huge number of hyaluronic acid based products on the market, some of which are derived from animals.

Collagen and Hyaluronic acid are both normal constituents of skin. Unfortunately they are slowly degraded by normal processes within the skin and are only a temporary solution to filling lines and tissue defects. The development of longer lasting tissue fillers is slightly more controversial. The substances used are often those not normally found within the skin structure. Therefore there is an increased risk of an allergic reaction, and there may not be a native degradation process within the tissue should problems occur. There are three permanent fillers with FDA approval at the time of writing, calcium hydroxyapatite microspheres, polylactic acid microspheres and polymethylmethacrolate microspheres.

The Uses of Fillers

Fillers are used to inject beneath fine lines and wrinkles on the face. They fill the skin beneath the line and make it less visible by removing the shadow it creates. They can also be used to correct the loss of volume in tissues, such as the lips, which will occur with increasing age. Fillers can be used to plump up areas of the face that have atrophied with age, creating a more youthful appearance.

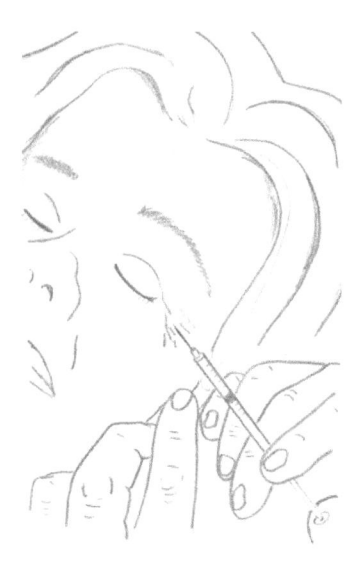

Topical anaesthetic (emla® cream) or cold packs applied to the skin are used for the injections. If treating the lips a nerve block with a local anaesthetic injection may be needed.

Types of Filler

There are two main types of Filler:

1. **Temporary Fillers**
2. **Permanent Fillers**

The most common fillers used are:

- **Collagen**
- **Hyaluronic acid**
- **Fat**

1. Temporary Fillers

Collagen Fillers

Collagen Filler	Source	FDA approval
Zyderm® *Zyplast*®	Collagen from cow's skin	Wrinkles, lines, scars.
Autologen®	Collagen from patient's skin	Wrinkles, lines, scars.
CosmoDerm® *CosmoPlast*®	Collagen from donated human skin	Wrinkles, lines, scars.
Cymetra®	Collagen from donated human skin	Wrinkles, lines, scars.
Isologen®	Collagen producing cells from patient's skin	Wrinkles, lines, scars.

Collagen has been available for injection since 1977 as Zyderm® (Allergan, Irvine, Calif). Zyplast® was then developed as a more robust product by cross-linking the collagen. These were the first widely used commercially available fillers. They consist of bovine (cow) collagen which is highly purified. They are used for smoothing lines, wrinkles, scars, and for defining the lip border. They last for four to six months. A skin test must be administered 4 weeks prior to treatment to screen for any pre-existing allergy to bovine collagen. Allergic reactions to bovine collagen have been reported in about three percent of patients.

Autologen® (Autogenesis Technologies, Acton, Mass) was the first human derived collagen to be produced commercially. It is derived from small pieces of the patients own skin, which are processed and prepared for injection. There is no risk of allergy as the tissue is derived from the recipient, but the production process is laborious and expensive. Human derived collagen is now also available from donor sources. Products include CosmoDerm® and CosmoPlast® (Allergan, Santa Barbara, Calif). These are human derived equivalents to Zyderm® and Zyplast® which the manufacturers claim do not require skin testing as there is no risk of allergy. CosmoDerm® 1 and 2 are used for fine lines and wrinkles, whilst CosmoPlast® is more robust and is used for deeper lines and folds. They were approved by the FDA in 2003. Clinical studies of injections with human collagen showed that the frequency of adverse immune responses (rejection by the body) with the use of CosmoDerm® 1 Human-Based Collagen is less than 1.3%.

Cymetra® (LifeCell Corporation, Palo, Calif) is another human derived collagen filler. It is made from micronized AlloDerm®, an acellular cadaveric dermis.

A novel approach to producing a filler comes in the form of Isologen® (Isologen technologies, Paramus, NJ). This product is produced by harvesting the skin cells form a small skin sample removed from the patient. The cells are then grown in culture and when sufficient numbers have been produced they are re-injected into the recipient. It is believed that as well as having a temporary filling effect the cells will produce new collagen within the skin, improving its quality and appearance.

Hyaluronic Acid Fillers

Hyaluronic Acid Fillers	Source	FDA approval
Restylane®	Hyaluronic acid from non-animal source	Wrinkles around nose and mouth
Restylane Fine-lines®	Hyaluronic acid from non-animal source	Not approved, used outside US
Perlane®	Hyaluronic acid from non-animal source	Moderate to severe facial folds and wrinkles
Juvaderm® *(24HV, 30, 30HV)*	Hyaluronic acid from non-animal source	Wrinkles and lines
Hylaform®	Hyaluronic acid from Rooster combs	Wrinkles around nose and mouth
Captique®	Hyaluronic acid from non-animal source	Wrinkles around nose and mouth

Hyaluronic acid has been available as Restylane® (Medicis, Scttsdale, Ariz) since 1996, and was FDA approved in 2003. There are three products available. Restylane® Touch is used for thin superficial lines, such as worry lines, and fine lines around the eyes and mouth. Restylane® Pure is used for deeper wrinkles such as those around the top of the nose (the glabella lines) and at the corners of the mouth (marionette lines). Restylane Perlane® is thicker and can be used for cheek folds (the nasolabial folds) and to thicken lips and create a pout. Hyaluronic acid is degraded by the surrounding tissues over a period of four to six months. The lines will recur and further treatments are needed.

Restylane® was the first hyaluronic acid based product to be given FDA approval, but there is now a multitude of products available. Products can be derived from hyaluronic acid produced by bacteria or derived from animals. The rooster comb is the most commonly used animal source. The longevity of the hyaluronic acid in the skin depends on the degree of cross-linking and hence the thickness of the injected gel. Injections placed deeper within the tissue will also last for a shorter duration. A study of 100 patients using hyalauronic acid for wrinkles showed that 60% of the effect was still present at 1 year.

Fat as Filler

Fat can be removed from one part of the body and injected into another. The technique has been championed by Dr Sydney Coleman in New York. Fat grafting techniques can be used to rejuvenate and enhance all areas of the face including the nasolabial folds, marionette lines, brow, upper eyelids, temples and lips. The procedure relies on liposuction to harvest the fat, which is processed and re-injected using a non-traumatic technique. The fat will not produce any allergic reaction. Unfortunately some of the fat is re-absorbed over time. It is not clear what percentage re-absorbs, but it may be as much as seventy percent and the treatments may need repeating. However, some permanent improvement is achieved.

Fat grafting can be done under local anaesthetic but more commonly patients elect to have a general anaesthetic. The process of liposuction is described in a later chapter. The harvested fat is then re-injected into the area to be treated. Most surgeons will over-treat the area expecting some of the fat to be re-absorbed, so the area may appear very swollen at first. This will diminish over the next month.

2. Permanent/ Semi-permanent Fillers

Longer lasting Fillers	Content	FDA approval
Radiesse®	Microspheres of calcium hydroxyapatite (coral) suspended in an aqueous gel carrier	Moderate to severe wrinkles and folds
Sculptra®	Synthetic polyactic acid in microspheres	Lipoatrophy only
ArteFill®	Polymethyl-methacrolate microspheres, bovine collagen gel and lignocaine	Correction of nasolabial folds

Radiesse® (BioForm Mediacal, San Mateo, Calif) contains microspheres of calcium hydroxyapatite which are 25 microns in diameter. Calcium hydroxyapatite is a normal constituent of bone and teeth. It is postulated that these microspheres persist after injection and new collagen is laid down around them. The effects are said to last for greater than one year, after which time the microspheres are degraded. There is no evidence that bone formation or nodules occur within the skin. Some surgeons have reservations over the injection of bone constituents or acrylic materials such as methylmethacrylate into the soft tissue of the face. When using long lasting tissue fillers any adverse events will, by definition, take longer to resolve and may be permanent. Patients should be fully aware of these risks.

Injection Techniques

There are four basic techniques for injecting fillers.

1. Serial puncture

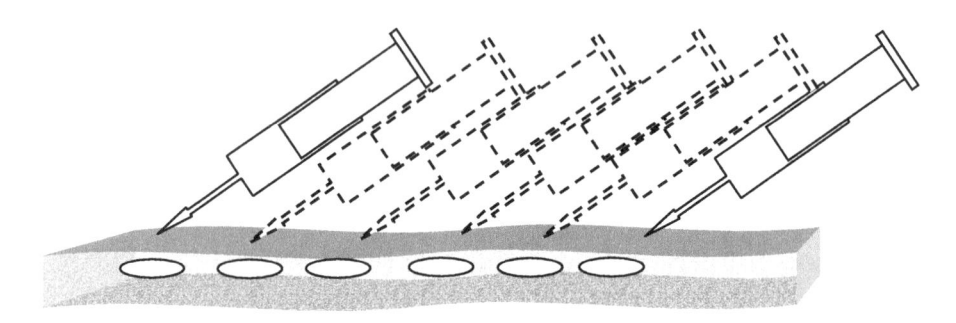

2. Linear threading

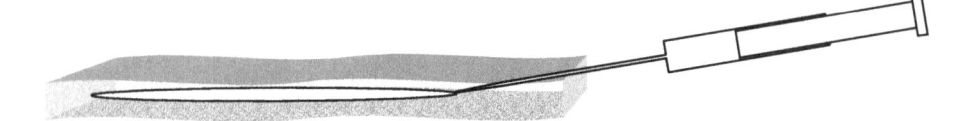

Fillers

3. Fanning

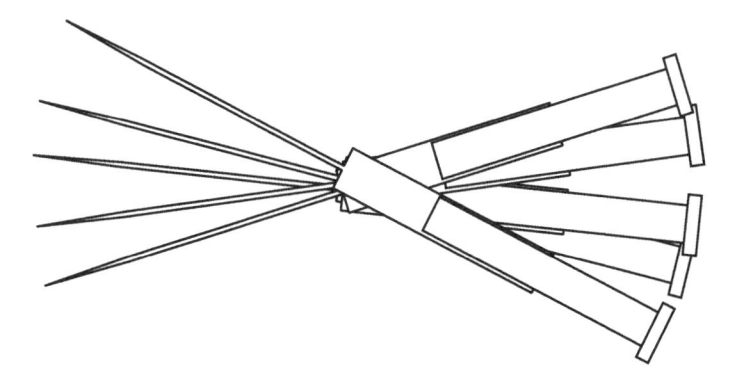

4. Cross-hatching

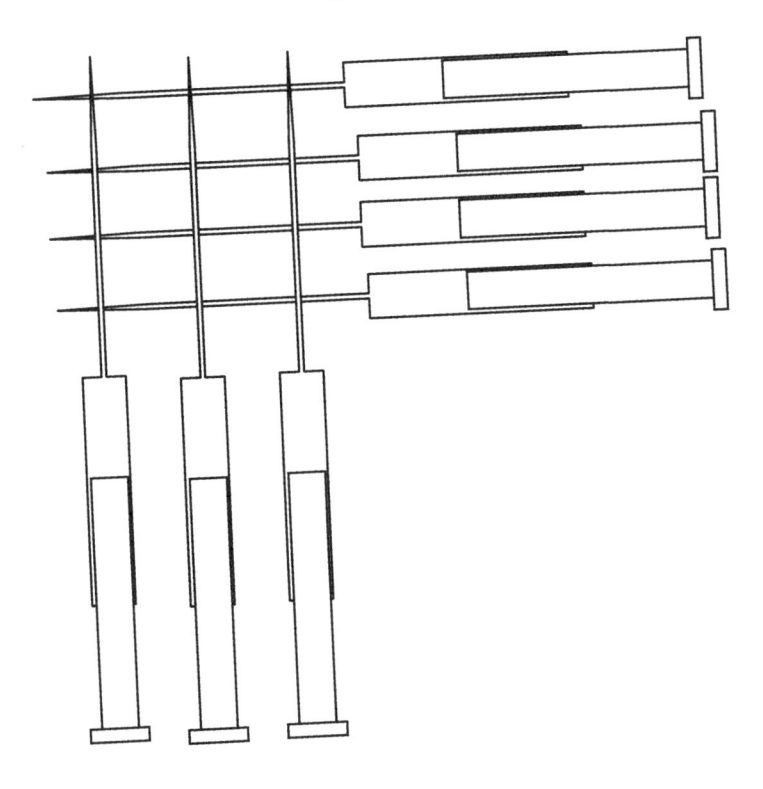

Facial Regions Commonly Treated with Fillers

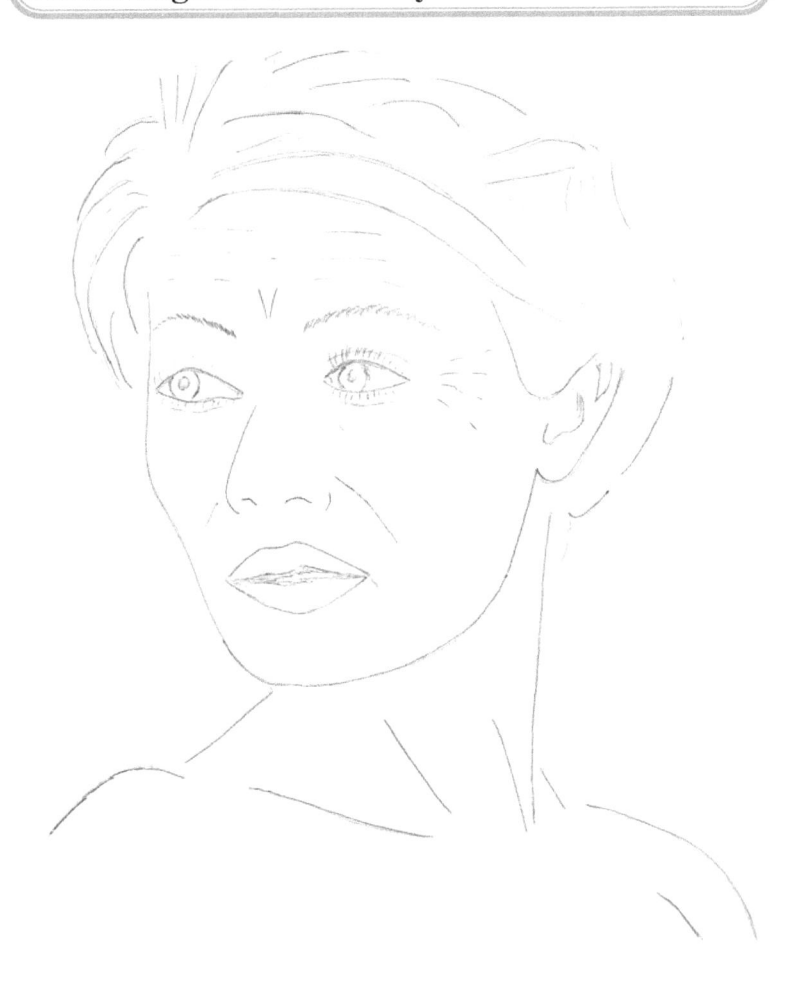

Glabella Lines

These can be treated using 0.5mls of hyaluronic acid injected into the mid-dermis using a serial puncture technique. The longevity of the result can be increased using concomitant Botox®.

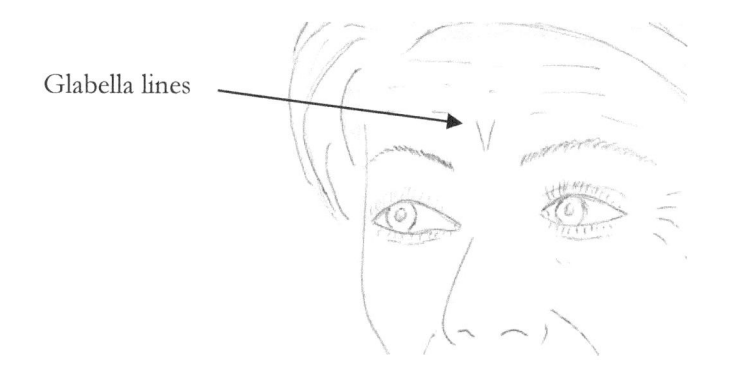

Glabella lines

Some authors recommend pressure on the supratrochlear vessels with the non-dominant hand during injection to reduce the risk of intravascular injection and bruising.

Forehead Lines

This area is best treated with hyaluronic acid using the linear threading or cross-hatching technique. The volume needed depends on the number and depth of the folds. Botox will make the hyaluronic acid last longer.

Crow's Feet around the Eyes

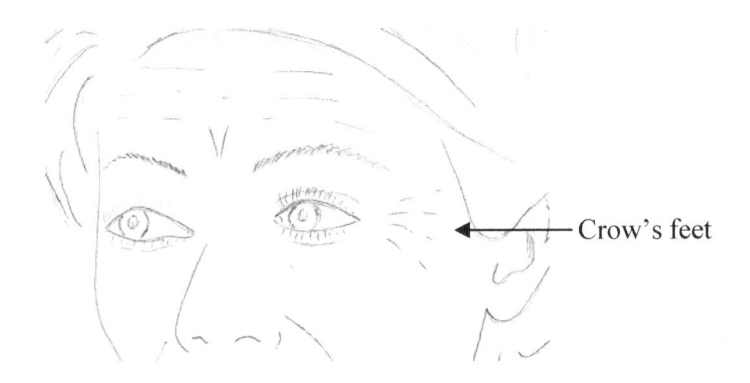

Crow's feet

The lines around the eye are often very fine and can be treated with small-particle hyaluronic acid injection at the dermal-epidermal level.

Nasolabial Fold

A combination of serial puncture and linear threading in the deep to mid-dermis is used in this region.

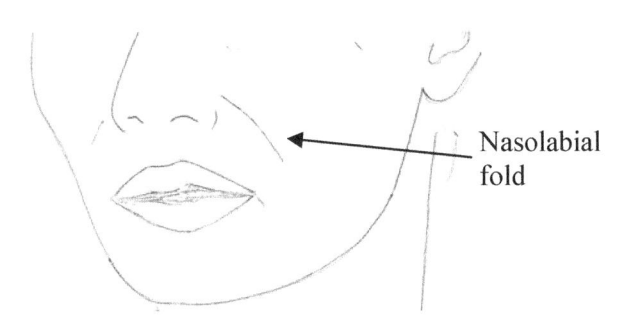

Nasolabial fold

Beginning near the lip and moving upwards, about 0.5 to 1 mls of larger particle hyaluronic acid is used each side. Alternatively, fat injections are effective in this region. It is important to avoid complete blunting of the fold, especially in the upper third as mobility and softness in this region conveys youthfulness.

Lips and Marionette Lines

Lip augmentation is a commonly requested cosmetic procedure, even in younger patients. In older patients the lips atrophy and become thinner. Vertical lines form around the lips and Marionette lines form at the corners of the mouth. These create a downturned appearance to the lips at rest, giving the impression of unhappiness.

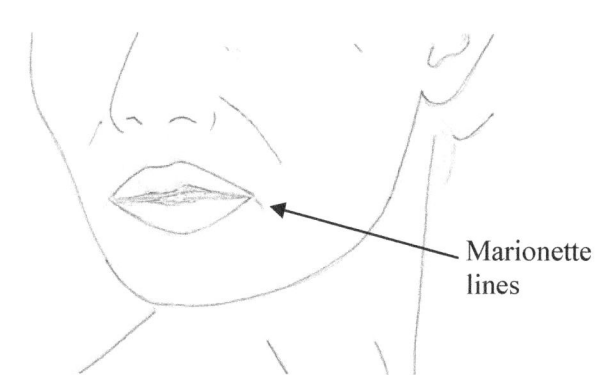

Marionette lines

Fat or hyaluronic acid can be used in the lips with good effect. One to 2 mls of fat can be placed in the upper and lower lip. The upper lip should be fullest centrally and at the corners of the mouth, whereas the lower lip should be fullest either side of the midline. Fat graft can produce bruising and swelling in the lips and the down time is slightly longer than with hyaluronic acid.

Younger patients will require enhancement of the lip-skin (vermillion-cutaneous) border, whilst older patients will also require volume replacement and filling of the marionette lines. These can be improved with hyaluronic acid used in a cross hatched pattern to fill the corners of the mouth. This can be enhanced with botox injection into the lip depressing muscle at the corner of the mouth (depressor anguli oris). Hyaluronic acid is then placed into the lip staring from the corner of the mouth. A serial puncture or linear threading technique is used to place the hyaluronic acid into the submucosal level, within the superficial orbicularis muscle (0.5 to 1.5mls per lip).

Contraindications to Fillers

Fillers should not be used if a patient has a history of anaphylaxis (severe allergy) from any cause, previous sensitivity to bovine collagen, lidocaine sensitivity, pregnancy or active infection at the treatment site. Caution should be used in anyone with a history of keloid or hypertrophic scar formation. Exposure of the treated area to excessive sun and extreme cold weather should be minimized until any initial swelling and redness have resolved.

Patients who are using substances that can prolong bleeding, such as aspirin or ibuprofen, as with any injection, may experience increased bruising or bleeding at injection site.

Adverse Effects of Fillers

Redness, swelling and bruising around the injection site are the most commonly seen adverse effects. These will usually resolve within the first week. Occasionally a more severe allergic reaction can develop. This occurs in about 3% of cases when bovine collagen is used, but less than 1% with other temporary fillers. Severe allergy can lead to skin breakdown and scarring, though this is rare. Small nodules can also form within or beneath the skin as a result of a more insidious allergic reaction. These nodules are rare, occurring in less than one percent of cases, but may be difficult to treat.

Over-treatment can cause lumpiness, persistent swelling and asymmetry. This can sometimes be reduced with massage. Over- injection of hyaluronic acid can sometimes be treated with hyaluronidase injection (an enzyme that breaks down hyaluronic acid).

There are about 120 different fillers available worldwide. The safety profile of many of them remains untested and their use is un-regulated in some countries.

INJECTABLE FILLERS	
Cost	UK: £150 - £800 US: $500 - $1500
Anaesthetic	Hyaluronic acid - nil Collagen - nil Fat – general or local anaesthetic
Hospital stay	Nil
Recovery	1 day
Risks	Bruising (transient) Redness Allergic reaction Over-treatment – swelling

3. Facial Peels

Who benefits from a facial peel?

A facial peel involves treating the face with a variety of substances which remove the most superficial layers of the skin. These will then regenerate. It will improve the quality of the skin, removing fine lines and improving irregular pigmentation. Facial peels vary in strength. Glycolic acid, trichloroacetic acid (TCA) and phenol are all used, the latter agents being stronger. Stronger peels will have a greater effect, but also carry increased risks of side effects. Light peels can be purchased from chemist shops and applied at home. Stronger peels must be applied by a dermatologist or plastic surgeon.

What does a facial peel involve?

Many doctors will use pre-treatment agents to prepare the skin prior to peeling. Pre-treatment with

Retin-A will help dekeratinize the skin surface to allow deeper and more even penetration for the peeling agent. 4% hydroquinone is a skin bleaching agent which is used to help reduce the skin pigment prior to peeling. This may help diminish the unwanted de-pigmentation produced by chemical peels. Retin-A and hydroxyquinine may be used for up to six weeks before the actual peel. The peel is not painful so it is done without anaesthetic. Light sedation is sometimes used. The surgeon will cover the patient's eyes and then apply the peeling agent using swabs or cotton wool balls.

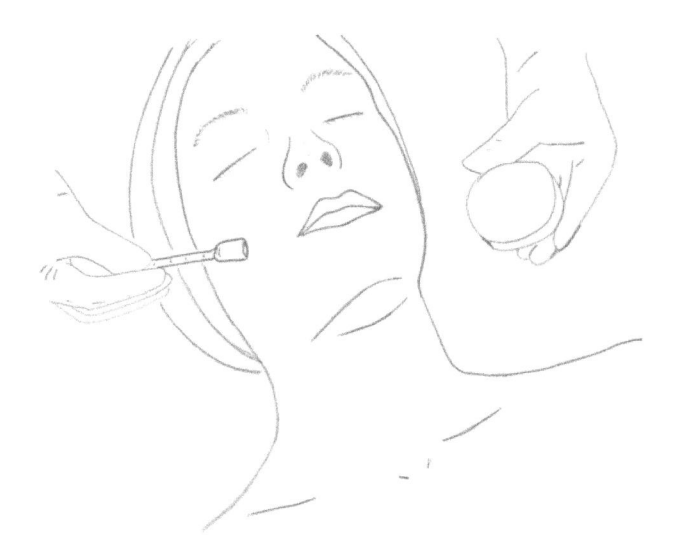

There may be an initial sting, but this will resolve quickly. The application process takes only about fifteen minutes for TCA peels but about two hours for a phenol peel. Patients will not need to stay in hospital overnight, but they should have someone to take them home. TCA and phenol peels will produce significant redness, swelling and some scaling of the skin. This will take about two weeks to resolve and patients may not wish to go out in public during this period. It is very important to avoid sun exposure and use sunscreen for several months after the procedure. The ultraviolet light in sunshine will cause burning and irregular pigmentation changes.

The improvements in skin quality will be mild with glycolic acid and will not be long lasting. TCA peels produce a more noticeable effect and will last longer, whilst phenol peels will have the most dramatic improvement with a long lasting result. The skin will continue to age at its normal rate.

What are the risks of facial peels?

A facial peel removes the most superficial layers of skin, but if the concentration of the agent is too strong, or is applied for too long, it removes the deeper skin layers. This can cause complications. The main risks from all peels are scarring, skin discoloration (hypopigmentation) and allergic reactions. Products purchased over the counter act very slowly, rarely produce scarring or skin pigment changes, but can provoke allergic reactions such as superficial irritation, redness and flaking. These are usually reversible. The improvements noticed from these products are variable. They will not be as good as stronger peels using TCA or Phenol.

TCA peel is used in various strengths and is often used in association with a blue dye to aid even application. It gives a medium depth peel which, when used in concentrations below 35%, has few complications. However, if applied in several coats it can produce a deeper skin peel with a greater risk of scarring and pigment changes.

Phenol peels can be done only under very close medical supervision. It creates a much deeper peel than other agents and historically was one of the first agents to be used. It is one of the few agents which will improve coarse wrinkles. However, it has a higher chance of producing scarring, and is almost always associated with some loss of skin pigmentation in the treated areas. It should not be used in dark skinned individuals. Phenol can be used only for small areas at a time and should be used only on the face as it may produce scarring if used on the neck. It should be avoided in people who have heart problems as it can cause irregularities of the heart beat.

A chemical peel produces an open skin wound over the area treated. As with any open wound, there is a risk of infection during the healing process. Antibiotics and anti-viral agents can be used to reduce this threat (especially if patients have had cold sores in the past).

FACIAL PEELS	
Cost	UK: £300 - £2,000 US: $500 - $5,000
Anaesthetic	nil
Hospital stay	nil
Recovery	**Glycolic acid - 1 day** (needs repeating regularly) **TCA - 7 to 10 days** (needs repeating annually) **Phenol – 10 to 21 days** (long lasting results)
Risks	**Redness** **Scarring** **Skin infection** **Skin pigment changes**

4. Laser

The Cosmetic Uses of Laser

Laser can be used for skin rejuvenation and correction of some skin blemishes. There are several types of laser commonly used for cosmetic surgery. The main uses are:

- Skin resurfacing and wrinkle ablation
- Hair removal
- Birthmark removal
- Tattoo removal
- Thread vein removal

The type of laser used for each of these differs, but they all act in a similar manner. They deliver a pulse of energy to the target tissue, causing localised destruction of that specific tissue. A specific laser will target a specific tissue.

Laser Skin Resurfacing

Lasers used for skin resurfacing include the carbon dioxide laser and the erbium laser.

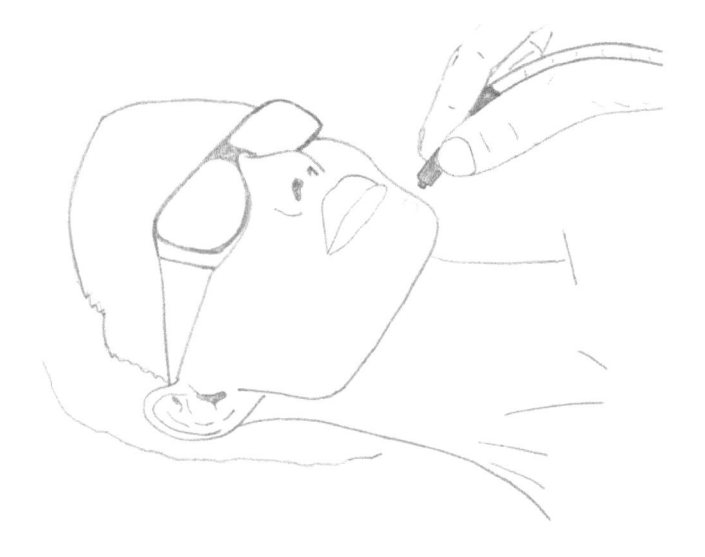

How does laser skin resurfacing work?

The carbon dioxide and erbium lasers vaporise the superficial layer of skin. The depth of skin vaporisation depends on the power of the laser and the number of passes used over the skin. The aim of treatment is to vaporise the superficial layers without destroying the full thickness of the skin. This allows the skin to regenerate from the deeper layers, removing skin blemishes and wrinkles. There is also some skin tightening associated with this process, this is probably due to changes in the skin collagen content. The speed of regeneration depends on the depth of skin vaporization. Deeper damage will take longer to heal. If the full thickness of the skin is accidentally vaporized then the resulting wound will heal by scar formation rather than skin regeneration.

Erbium and carbon dioxide lasers will improve wrinkles, sun damaged skin and some acne scars. They can improve the appearance of scars and help tighten slack facial skin. They will not improve fine veins over the face, known as telangiectasia or spider veins. These require a pulsed dye or KTP laser.

What does laser skin resurfacing involve?

Laser skin resurfacing is done under a general anaesthetic. It is too painful to be done awake, especially if the whole face is to be treated. Most people will go home the next day. The laser creates a superficial burn over the area treated. This is painful, so patients will often need analgesics for a few days.

The appearance of this burn is often very alarming, especially if patients are uninformed. This is the typical result and normal mechanism of the treatment. The burn will heal over the next two weeks. Some surgeons give their patients antibiotics and antiviral agents. This reduces the risk of bacterial infections or an outbreak of herpes in patients who get cold sores.

After a couple of weeks the skin is usually healed but often remains red for a further month or two. Make up can be used as soon as the treated area is healed.

What are the risks of laser treatment?

Laser resurfacing is a safe procedure in experienced hands. It avoids the risk of bleeding problems or nerve damage which can be encountered with a surgical facelift. However, laser skin resurfacing will not address many of the ageing problems which can be treated with a surgical face lift, such as excess chin fat, and sagging jowls.

Like any procedure, laser skin resurfacing is associated with specific risks. Unfortunately there is a fine balance between getting no improvement, good improvement and skin damage. If the laser is set on a high power setting or passed too many times, there is a risk of skin damage. The wound can take more than three weeks to heal, and when it does the skin becomes red and lumpy in the over-treated areas. Skin damage is most common in areas where the skin is very thin, such as around the eyes or the lips. This type of scarring is rare. However, it can be devastating if it occurs.

Patients with dark skin are at risk of permanent skin pigment changes. This is due to the destruction of the pigment producing cells, causing skin pallor. Likewise, pale skinned patients who do not protect their skin from the sun after laser surgery are at risk of increased pigmentation.

As with any open wound, there is a risk of infection during the healing process. This can be from bacteria or the herpes virus. Infections usually respond to treatment with antibiotics and acyclovir, an antiviral agent. However, infection does increase the risk of scarring.

LASER SKIN RESURFACING	
Cost	UK: £1,000 - £3,000 US: $2,500 – 5,000
Anaesthetic	General
Hospital stay	Overnight
Recovery	14 - 21 days
Risks	Redness (can last up to 6 months) Scarring Skin infection Skin pigment changes (increased or decreased)

Laser Hair Removal

Lasers used for hair removal include the Ruby laser, Alexandrite laser, Nd YAG laser and Intense Pulsed Light source (IPL- not strictly a laser).

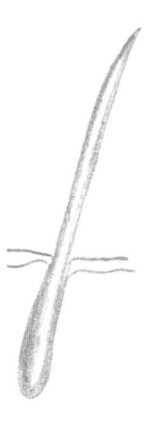

How does laser hair removal work?

The lasers target melanin which lies within the base of hair follicles. They deliver enough energy to selectively destroy the melanin collecting at the base of the hair, and hence eliminate further hair growth. Unfortunately, a single treatment will stop only a small proportion of the hair growth. Hair grows in cycles, and the laser is only capable of treating actively

Laser

growing hair (anagen phase hair). The resting phase for hair follicles (telogen phase hair) varies from six to twenty weeks, depending on the body region. This is why the laser treatment has to be repeated at six

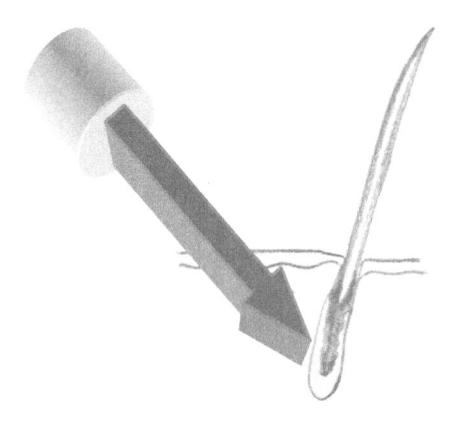

weekly intervals. Optimal hair removal will take between two to six sessions.

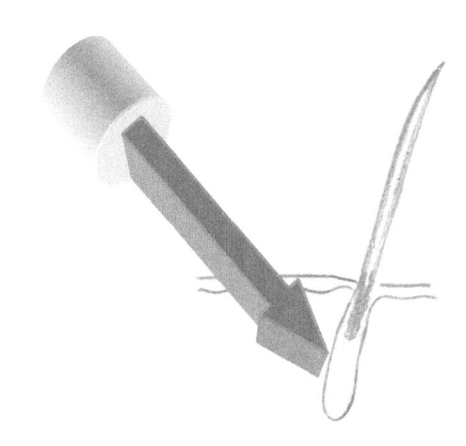

Skin around the hair also contains some melanin. The laser can also target this pigment causing unwanted effects, such as skin lightening or scarring. This can be reduced by using skin cooling devices during the laser treatment.

What does laser hair removal involve?

Laser hair removal only requires a local anaesthetic. The hair is shaved and a topical anaesthetic (e.g. emla cream) is applied. A cooling probe is often used, and this also helps to numb the area being treated. There is often some redness around the area after the procedure, but this diminishes over the next few days.

Laser hair removal is better at removing dark hair than fair hair. Skin pigment changes are more likely to occur in patients with dark skin.

LASER HAIR REMOVAL	
Cost	**UK: £150 - £400** **US: $300 - $800** **per treatment (up to six needed)**
Anaesthetic	**Topical local anaesthetic**
Hospital stay	**Nil**
Recovery	**Nil**
Risks	**Redness (lasts 2-7 days)** **Skin pigment changes** (increased or decreased) **Scarring (very rare)**

5. Facelift

A facelift is a procedure to rejuvenate the ageing face. As men and women get older, the skin stretches and loses its elasticity. This produces wrinkles and excess skin which can hang down as a jowl under the chin. The fat in your face will also sag with increasing age, and the face becomes thinner.

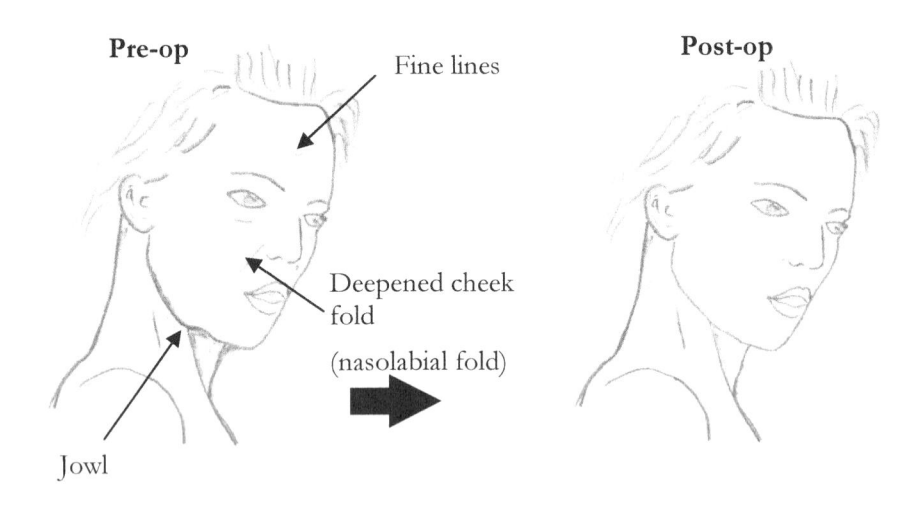

Pre-op — Fine lines, Deepened cheek fold (nasolabial fold), Jowl

Post-op

A facelift will remove this excess skin. At the same time the face is pulled upwards and backwards, correcting any sagging fat, giving a younger appearance. Stretching the skin also removes some of the facial wrinkles and fine lines.

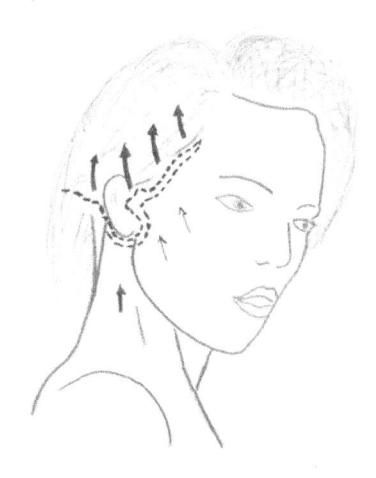

A facelift will not improve the fine lies in the forehead. This requires a brow lift or Botox injections. The fine lines around the eye may be improved by a facelift, but the excess skin in the upper eyelid and any lower eyelid "bags" will not change. These features of ageing will need a blepharoplasty to improve them.

What does a facelift involve?

The operation takes between 2 and 4 hours. It is done under a general anaesthetic. The surgeon makes a cut down the front of the ear, which then curls up behind the ear and then into or around the hairline towards the back of the head.

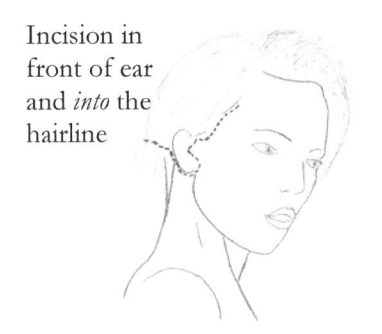

Incision in front of ear and *into* the hairline

Alternate incision in front of ear and *around* the hairline

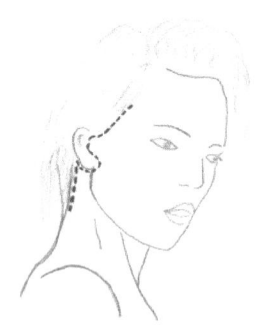

The surgeon then lifts the skin from the face and pulls it upwards and backwards, finally removing the excess skin.

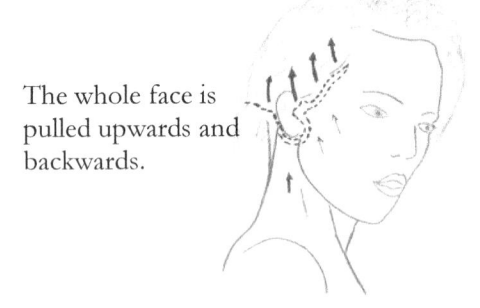

The whole face is pulled upwards and backwards.

The wound is then sutured. When the patient wakes up they will have a drain in each side. This is a small tube the size of a drinking straw, attached to a small bottle. This is usually removed the following day by a nurse on the ward. It is relatively painless.

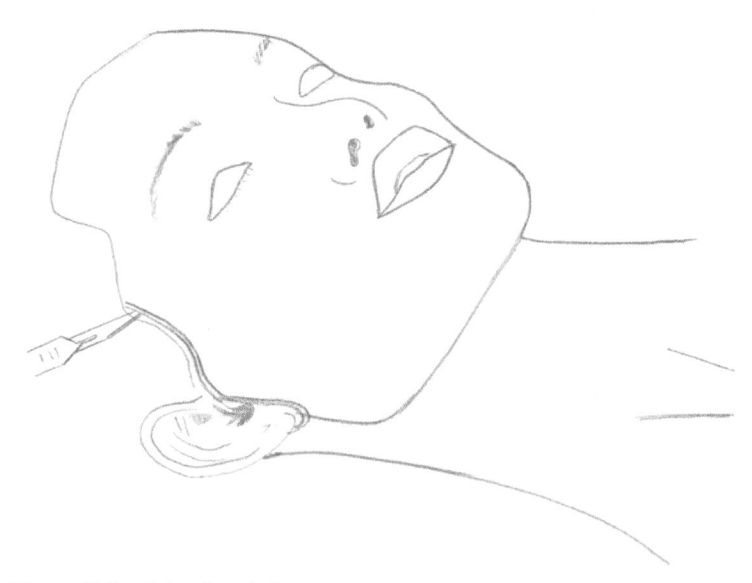

Facelift skin incision

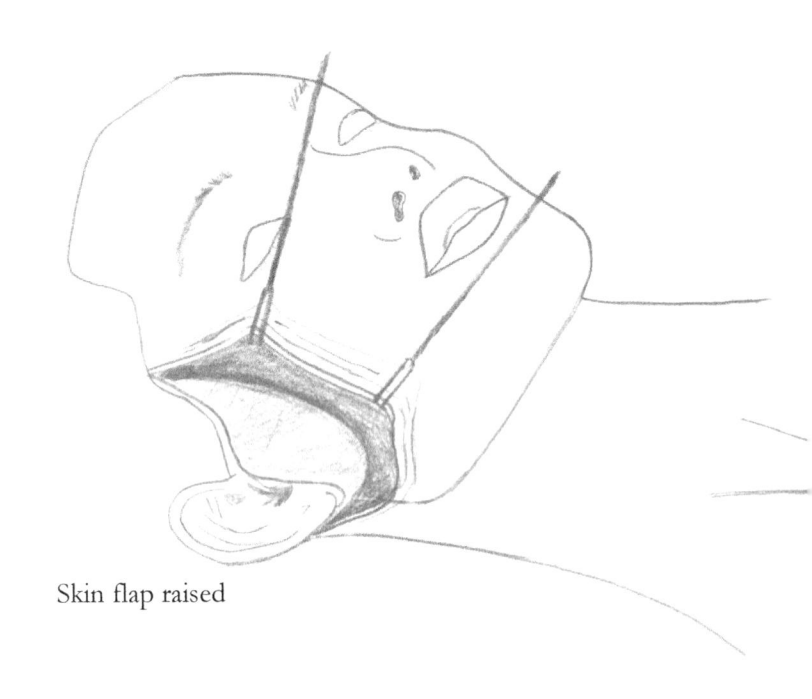

Everybody's Guide to Cosmetic Plastic Surgery

Skin flap raised

Excess skin excised

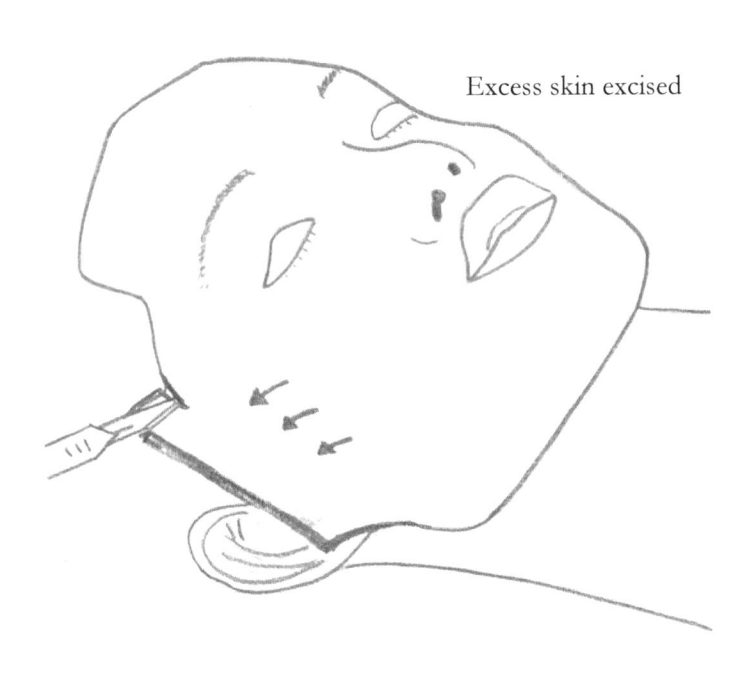

The day after surgery the patients face will be swollen, and this swelling will not go down for a few days. If all goes well, patients will be in hospital for a couple of days, then allowed home. Some surgeons bandage the face up for a few days, but this is done less commonly now. Most patients will not wish to go out much for a couple of weeks, mainly due to the swelling and bruising, but this will improve with time. The sutures will be removed within the first week, again a relatively painless procedure. The wounds heal within the first two weeks. Vigorous physical activity should be limited for several weeks, including jogging, bending, heavy housework, sex, or any activity that increases blood pressure. The scar will start to become less red after about six to eight weeks, but it will not truly settle down into a fine white scar for a year or so. It is important to avoid sun exposure for several months till the scars have matured.

Types of Facelift

There are several types of facelift available. A surgeon will often have a preferred technique.

Subcutaneous facelift: This involves lifting the skin only. This operation does not produce the same longevity of results as other techniques and is rarely used now.

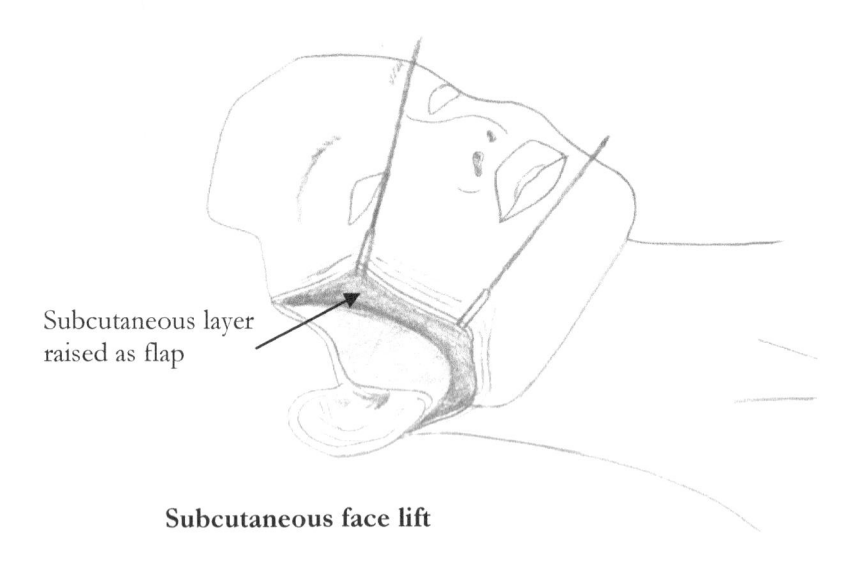

Subcutaneous layer raised as flap

Subcutaneous face lift

SMAS facelift: This is the technique used by most surgeons today. It involves lifting the skin and the layer directly beneath it (the SMAS). This deeper layer gives better support to the lift and longer lasting results than a simple subcutaneous lift.

SMAS facelift

Subcutaneous layer

SMAS layer

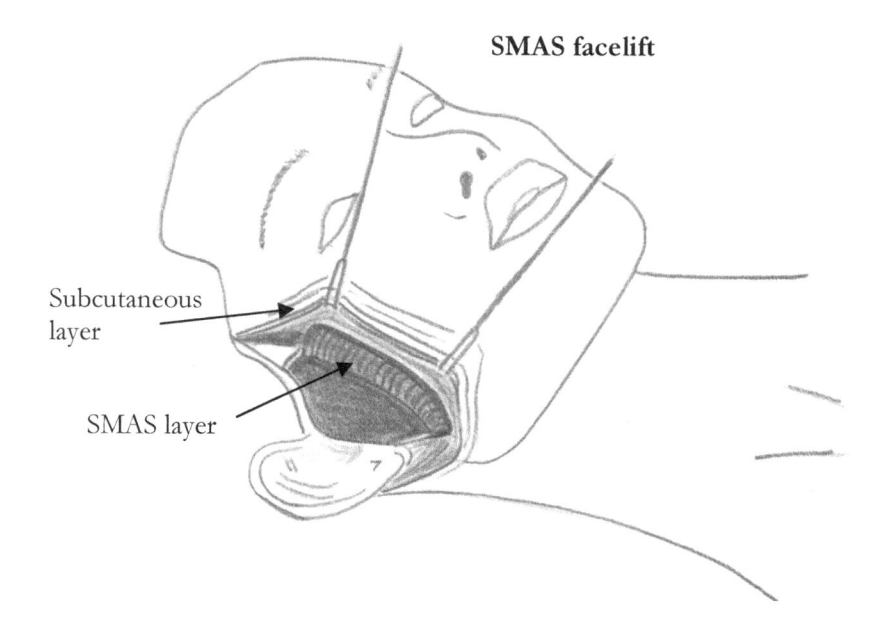

The SMAS layer is pulled upwards and backwards and sutured in this position to lift the rest of the face. The facial nerve lies directly beneath this layer and is at risk of damage or bruising. This can produce facial weakness.

MACS facelift: This technique involves a smaller incision. The skin is separated from the deeper layer and then three loops of suture material are used to hoist the SMAS layer upwards, producing the facelift.

MACS facelift

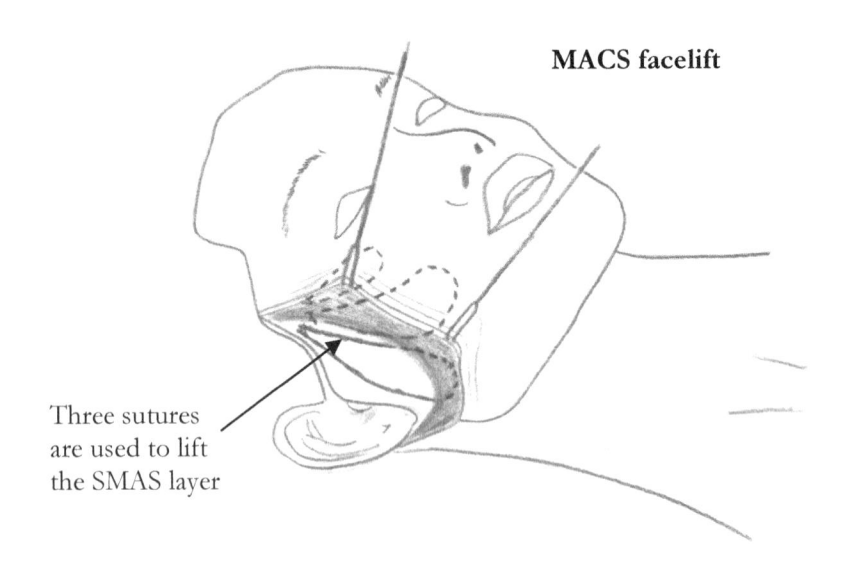

Three sutures are used to lift the SMAS layer

These techniques can be combined with a small incision in the neck just under the chin. This allows the muscles in the neck (the platysma) to be plicated (tightened). This lifts the neck. Fat can be removed from the neck through the same incision to improve the definition of the jaw-line.

What risks are involved with a facelift?

A facelift is a complex operation and there are a number of potential problems associated with the surgery. A percentage of patients (about five to ten percent) will get a small collection of blood forming under the skin within 24 hours of surgery (a haematoma). If this occurs another small procedure is needed to remove it, often needing a general anaesthetic. Patients who take aspirin are more prone to bleeding.

A small percentage of people will get a wound infection. This usually occurs after three or four days and makes the wound red and painful. It almost always improves with antibiotics. The scar usually fades into a fine line with time, but in some people this may not occur. A small percentage of patients will form a prominent scar which remains as a thick lumpy red line. This occurs more often in people with very pale skin and red hair. Younger people are also more prone to this. The scar can also stretch, leaving a wide pale scar. If you smoke or are diabetic you may have even worse problems with the scar. The blood supply to the skin is not as good and small areas of skin can die, leaving a very prominent scar on the cheek or behind the ear. Many surgeons will not perform a facelift on smokers for this reason.

The surgeon's incision will often go into the hairline both in front of and behind the ear. This can cause a couple of problems. An area of hair loss can develop around the scar. There may also be a small step in the hairline either side of the scar. This is often so minor that it is not noticeable to other people.

When the surgeon lifts the skin from the face there are several nerves which can be damaged. The most commonly injured nerve provides sensation to the ear. If it is damaged it will produce a numb ear. The earlobe is said to feel like it "belongs to someone else". The other nerves which can be damaged, though very rarely, supply the muscles which move the face. This can create an immobile forehead, with an eyebrow that you cannot raise. Likewise it may produce a slight droop on one side of the mouth with an asymmetric smile. Fortunately these nerve injuries are very rare, occurring in less than one percent of facelifts. Most of them recover over a period of three to six months.

Minor problems include strange sensations in the skin of the face, small lumps and asymmetries, but most of these improve with time.

FACELIFT	
Cost	UK: £ 4,000 - £8,000 US: $7,000 – $9,000
Anaesthetic	General Anaesthetic
Hospital stay	1 – 3 days
Recovery	14 - 28 days
Risks	Haematoma Redness Scarring Wound infection Skin pigment changes Asymmetry Nerve damage Earlobe numbness Skin contour changes Hair loss Hairline anomalies

6. Brow lift

Who benefits from a brow lift?

Age changes in the upper face include forehead lines, descent of the eyebrow and laxity of the upper eyelid skin. The upper eyelid develops excess skin which droops over the eye, producing a "tired" expression. Fine lines appear adjacent to the eyes, known as "crow's feet".

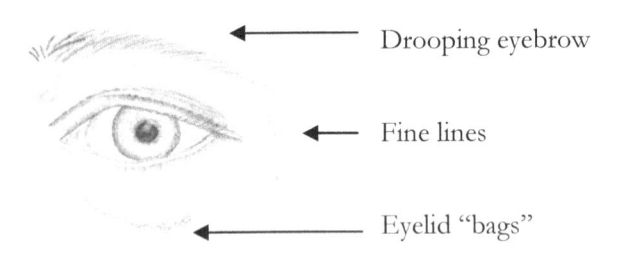

← Drooping eyebrow

← Fine lines

← Eyelid "bags"

A brow lift will improve the forehead lines and reposition the eyebrows.

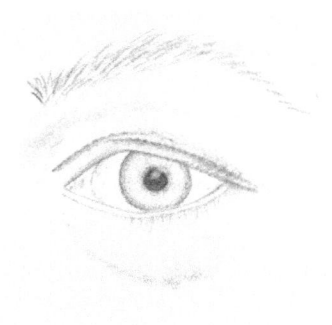

The upper eyelid laxity may be improved with a brow lift, but this often also needs an eyelid incision to fully correct it (a blepharoplasty). The "crow's feet" lines around the eye will be improved, especially when combined with a facelift procedure.

What is a brow lift?

The surgery aims to raise the eyebrows and remove forehead wrinkles. There are several techniques commonly used. The classic open brow lift involves making an incision across the top of the forehead in the hairline.

Coronal brow lift incision

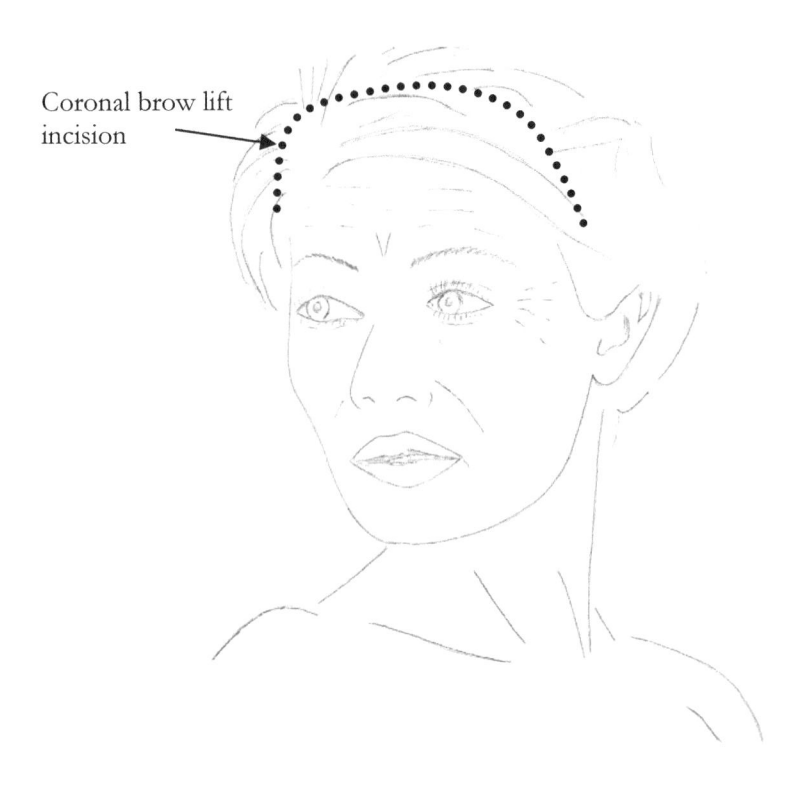

This is called a coronal incision. It follows the line of a pair of headphones across the top of the scalp. The entire forehead is lifted upwards, excising the excess skin. If the hairline is high or receding, the incision may be placed just at the hairline, to avoid adding even more height to the forehead.

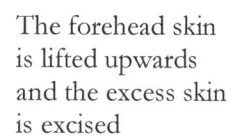

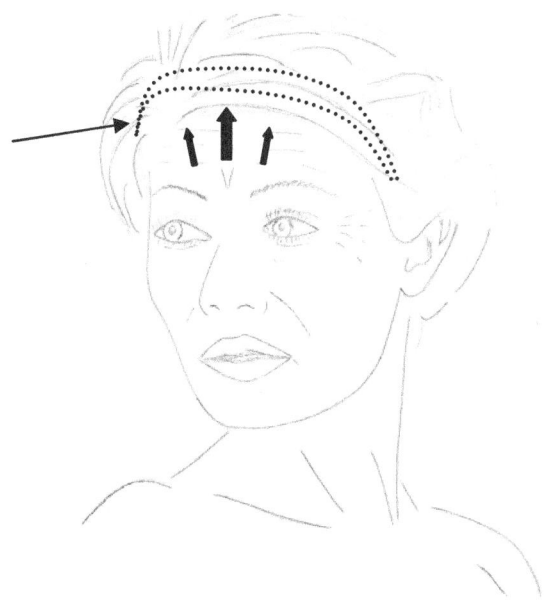

The forehead skin is lifted upwards and the excess skin is excised

The classic open technique is used less since the introduction of endoscopic brow lifts. This involves making several smaller incisions within the hairline. An endoscope (a miniature telescope with a camera) is then passed into the wound to create a space under the forehead, releasing its attachments to the underlying bone. The forehead is then lifted upwards and fixed in its new position with screws or specially designed grips. The screws need to be removed after about ten days, but the grips are re-absorbed by the tissues. Patients who are bald or who have a receding hairline benefit from this approach as the scars are less visible than those associated with the classic brow lift.

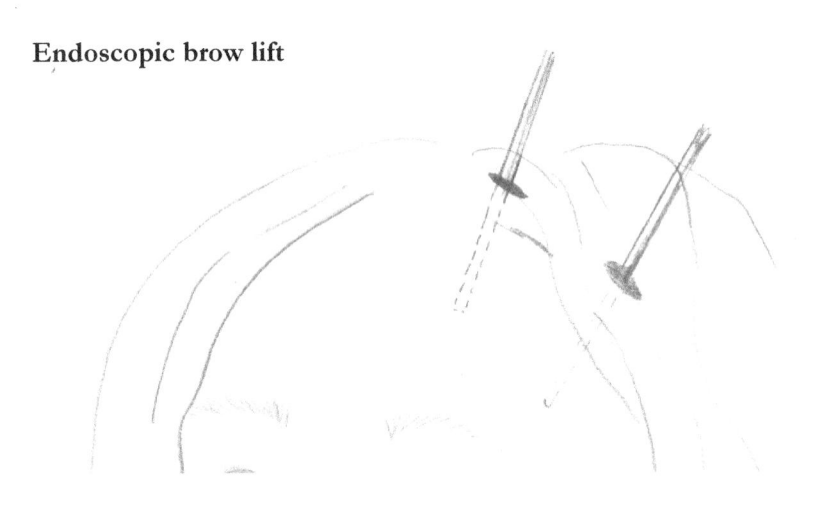

Endoscopic brow lift

Another technique which can be used in older patients is an open brow lift involving an incision just above the eyebrow. The advantage of this technique is that it can be done under local anaesthetic. It leaves a scar above the eyebrow but this is barely visible in older patients. It is not recommended for young patients who will often get a very prominent scar.

Open brow lift

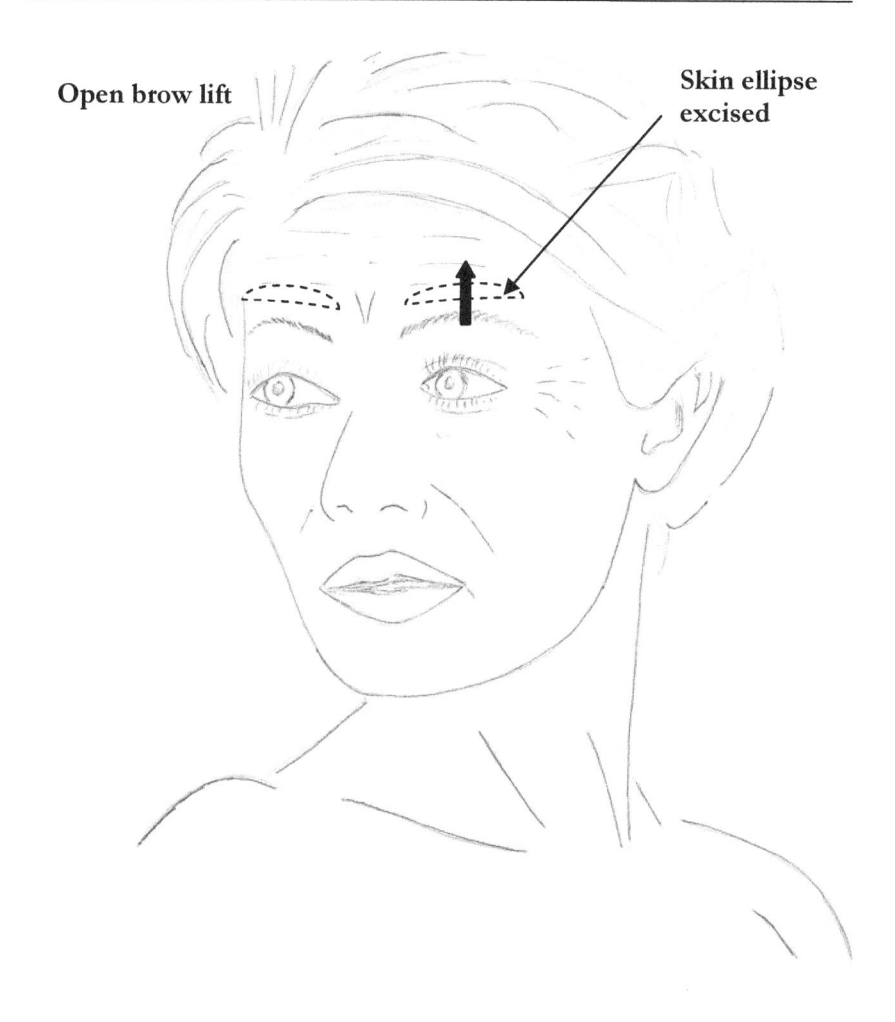

Skin ellipse excised

Recent innovations include the use of barbed threads to elevate the eyebrows. These are passed under the skin from the hairline to the eyebrow. They grip the tissue, lifting the brow. The procedure is less invasive compared to traditional brow lifts, but there is some risk of the sutures being extruded over time. Although results are promising more long term results are required before the technique can be recommended.

Thread lift

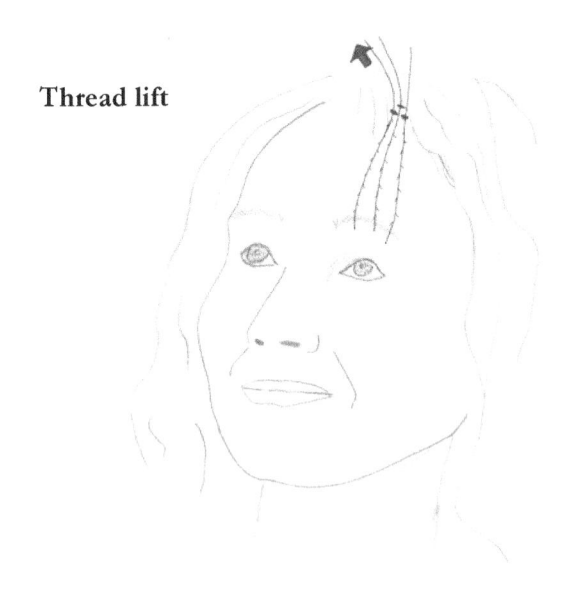

What does an endoscopic brow lift involve?

A brow lift is done under a general anaesthetic. The patient will go into hospital on the day of surgery. The surgeon and anaesthetist will review them before the procedure, and then they will be taken down to the operating theatre and put to sleep. The forehead is often very swollen after the surgery. There may be one or two small drains placed within the scalp. These are removed the following day. Patients usually go home the next day, but they will still have a swollen forehead and eyelids for a couple of weeks. Vigorous physical activity should be limited for several weeks, including jogging, bending, heavy housework, sex, or any activity that increases blood pressure. The scar from this operation is within the hairline and will fade over the course of 6 to 8 weeks, by which stage it is often barely visible.

What are the risks involved with brow lift surgery?

A percentage of patients (about five to ten percent) will get a small collection of blood forming under the skin within 24 hours of surgery. If this occurs another small procedure is needed to remove it, often needing a general anaesthetic. Patients who take aspirin are more prone to bleeding. A similar problem can develop at a later stage. This is called a seroma and is less common. It is due to a collection of serum within the wound and can sometimes be removed by aspiration with a needle and syringe rather than another operation.

Brow lift scars are hidden within the hairline, but sometimes a broad scar can form, leaving a strip of hairless skin within the scalp. This may be treated surgically by removing the wide scar tissue so that a finer scar develops. Sometimes hair loss develops along the scar edges. This usually grows back after a few months. Loss of sensation along or just beyond the incision line is common. It often resolves but may be permanent.

If bleeding complications occur during an endoscopic forehead lift, your surgeon may have to abandon the endoscopic approach and switch to the conventional, open procedure. This results in a more extensive scar and a longer recovery period.

ENDOSCOPIC BROW LIFT	
Cost	UK: £ 3,000 - £4,000 US: $3,500 – $5,000
Anaesthetic	General Anaesthetic
Hospital stay	Overnight
Recovery	14 days
Risks	**Wound infection** **Prominent scars** **Bleeding or haematoma** **Seroma** **High eyebrows** **Asymmetric eyebrows** **Forehead numbness** **Forehead itching** **Headaches** **Forehead paralysis**

7. Eyelid Surgery (Blepharoplasty)

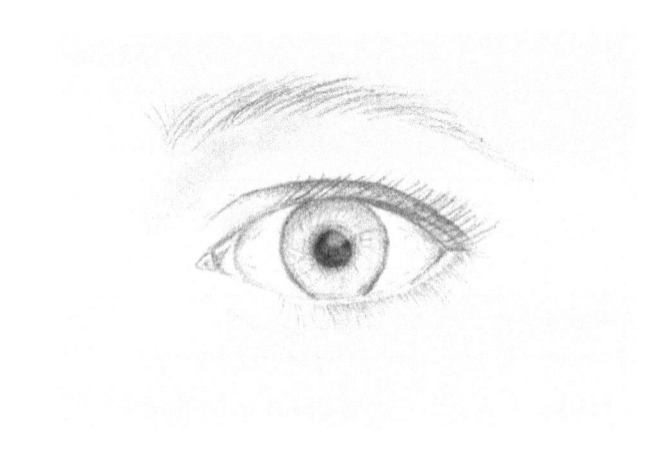

Who benefits from eyelid surgery?

Age brings on several changes in the eyelids. It can affect both upper and lower eyelids. The upper eyelid develops excess skin which droops over the eye, producing a "tired" expression. The lower eyelids often get "bags" under them. This is produced by fat around the eye bulging down and out and distorting the lower eyelid.

Blepharoplasty

Excess upper eyelid skin

Lower eyelid "bags"

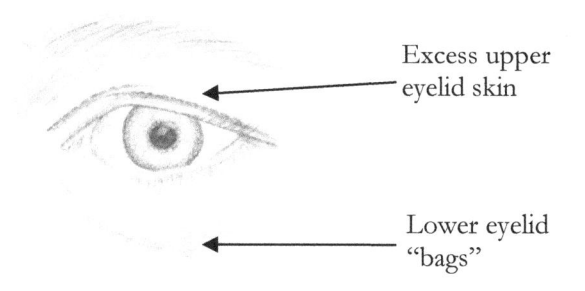

What does eyelid surgery aim to do?

The surgery aims to reduce this "tired" expression in the eyes by excising the extra skin from the upper eyelids and repositioning the fat in the lower eyelids. The skin incisions are shown below.

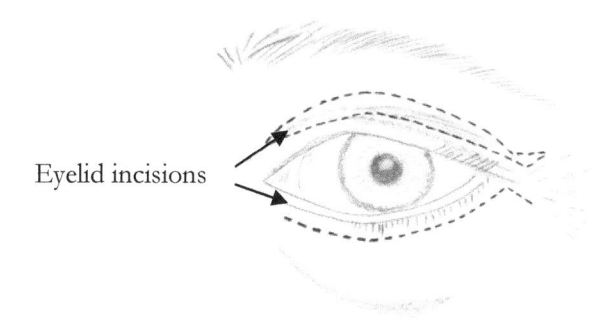

Eyelid incisions

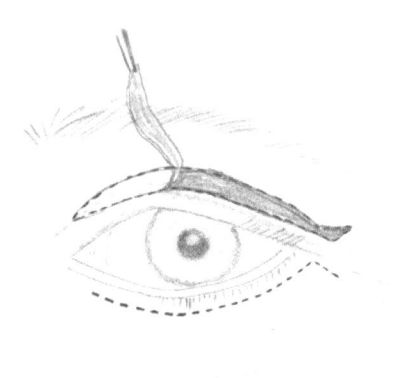

Sometimes the fat within the eyelids is excised, but this can create a "hollow eye" appearance. Some surgeons now reposition the fat rather than excise it.

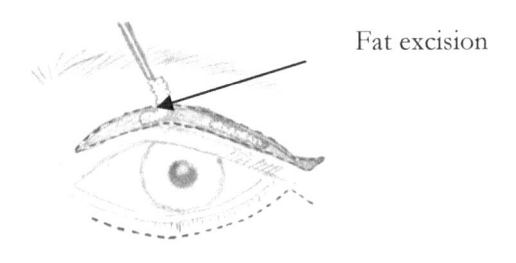

Fat excision

Laser eyelid surgery involves making an incision inside the lower eyelid with a laser. There is no visible scar on the lower eyelid. There may also be a reduced risk of bleeding complications as the laser coagulates blood vessels when it cuts through them.

Laser incision inside the lower eyelid

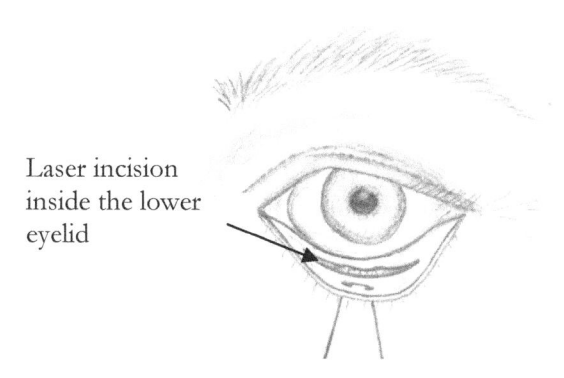

The disadvantage of laser eyelid surgery is that any excess skin can not be excised through the incision, therefore it is often not suitable for all patients.

What does the eyelid surgery involve?

Upper eyelid surgery can be done with a local anaesthetic injection. However, lower eyelid surgery always needs to be done under a general anaesthetic. Patients often go into hospital on the day of surgery. When they wake up the eyelids are often very swollen. The surgeon may put some cold packs over the eyes to help reduce the swelling. Patients usually go home the next day, but they will still have swollen eyelids for a couple of weeks. Vigorous physical activity should be limited for several weeks, including jogging, bending, heavy housework, sex, or any activity that increases blood pressure. Some surgeons use sutures that need to be removed after a week. This is a simple procedure which can be done in the outpatient clinic. The scar from this operation will fade over the course of 6 to 8 weeks, by which stage it is often barely visible.

What are the risks involved with eyelid surgery?

The operation is relatively safe. However, some problems can occur. Patients with thyroid problems, glaucoma, high blood pressure or dry eyes should probably avoid this type of cosmetic surgery. People who smoke are also more likely to have problems with poor wound healing. There are a few problems which can arise from eyelid surgery, even in the hands of the best surgeons. A small number of wounds will become infected (about one or two percent) thus needing a course of antibiotics. There will be a scar on each treated eyelid, and this can sometimes become lumpy, raised and red. This occurs more commonly in young people with fair skin, and it can be very noticeable.

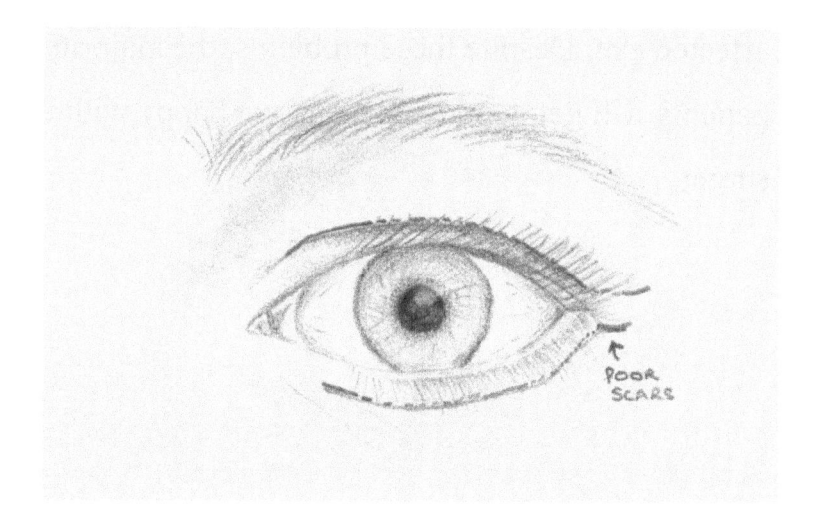

There is also a risk of removing too much or too little skin. Removing too little skin will result in the eyes still looking "tired", but the surgery can always be repeated after a settling down period. However, if too much skin is removed this can lead to difficulty in closing the eyes. This will often resolve after a couple of days, but very occasionally it requires further surgery to correct the problem. Other problems include asymmetry of the eyelids after surgery, corneal abrasions and dry eyes. Rarely, the muscles which move the eyes can be damaged, causing blurred or double vision. One very rare problem encountered with eyelid surgery is bleeding into the back of the eye socket. This probably occurs in only about 1 in a million operations, but it can cause blindness in the affected eye. Despite these problems, the majority of patients will get good results and are happy with the surgery.

EYELID SURGERY (BLEPHAROPLASTY)	
Cost	UK: £ 3,000 - £4,000 US: $4,000 – $5,500
Anaesthetic	General Anaesthetic
Hospital stay	Overnight
Recovery	14 days
Risks	Wound infection Prominent scars Bleeding Dry eyes Asymmetry Inverted eyelashes Hollow eye appearance Raised eye pressure (glaucoma – rare) Eyelid droop (ptosis) Double vision (rare) Loss of vision (rare)

8. Nose Surgery (Rhinoplasty)

Who benefits from nose surgery?

The shape of the nose is very variable. Men and women have different nasal features. Men tend to have larger noses which are broader and longer.

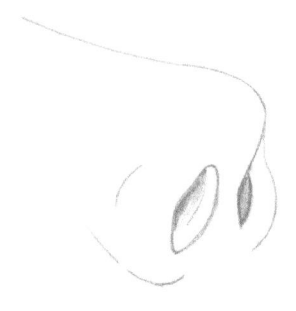

Some people are born with a hump on their noses, while others will injure their nose through sport or fights. Traumatic nasal injuries can be pushed back straight if they are treated within a week. If the nasal deviation is not corrected within this time frame then it has to be re-broken to correct the deformity. Re-shaping of the nose is called a rhinoplasty.

The appearance of the nose is related to the shape of the chin and forehead. A small chin will make a nose look larger. A sloped forehead will make a nose look longer.

When considering nasal surgery patients will need to decide what they dislike about their nose. There are several common problems. The most common is a hump on the bridge of the nose. This is relatively easy to correct.

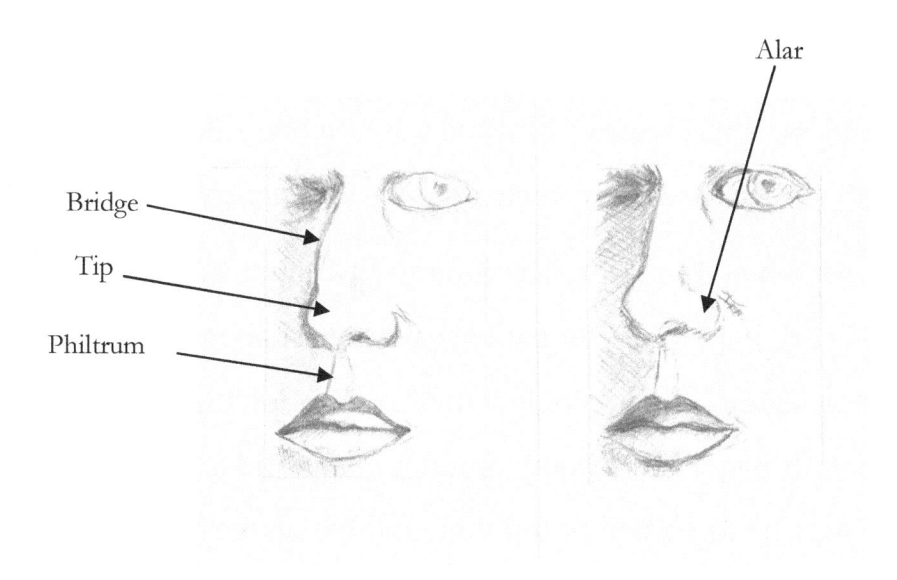

Alar

Bridge
Tip
Philtrum

The problem can also be within the tip of the nose. This may be too broad (a bulbous nose) or it may be too small (a pinched nose). This can be corrected, but it is slightly more challenging for the surgeon.

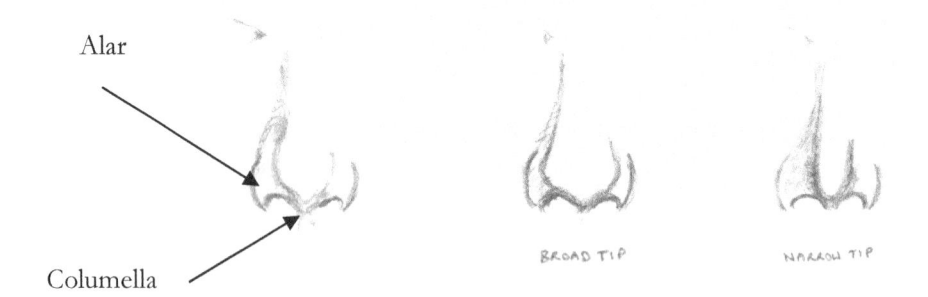

Alar

Columella

BROAD TIP

NARROW TIP

Patients may also have problems inside the nose, in the airway. This is caused by a deviation in the septum (the wall inside the nose between the two nostrils). This creates a blocked nose on one side or both. It can also be corrected during the surgery.

When discussing nasal surgery with the surgeon it is very important that patients are honest about what bothers them. They may feel their nose is too big or too small. It may have a hump or a dip in the bridge. The tip may be too broad or too thin, and the tip may hang down or point up too much. The patient's description of the problem will help the surgeon plan the surgery. They will listen to what the patient says, and then tell them how surgery can help.

Most of the time the surgeon will agree with the patient, but sometimes they may think the problem is too small to have a good chance of correcting it.

How is a rhinoplasty done?

A rhinoplasty (nose job) can be performed either "closed" or "open". The first technique leaves all the scars on the inside of the nose.

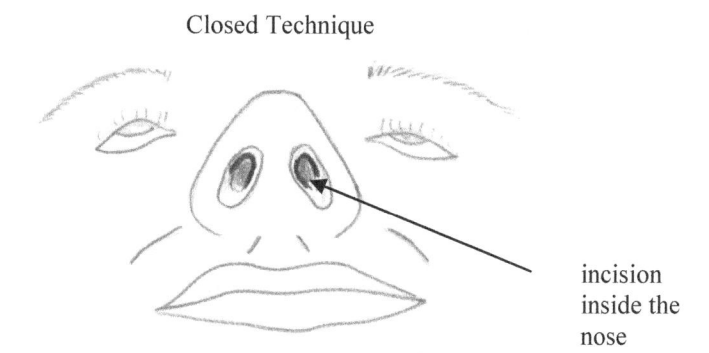

Closed Technique

incision inside the nose

The "open" technique leaves a small scar on the columella (the bit between your nostrils). The surgery can often be done using either technique, and it depends on the preference of the operating surgeon.

Open Technique

incision in the columella

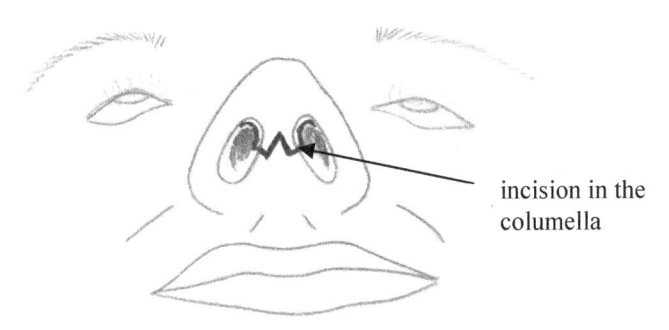

Significant changes to the tip of the nose are more commonly performed using the "open" technique with a small visible scar. These scars are usually not noticeable after a few months.

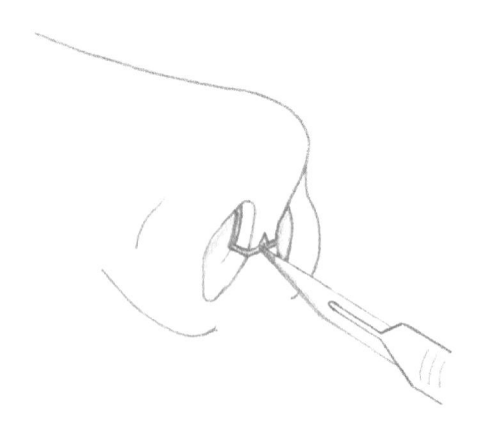

The operation begins by making an incision in the nose. The skin is then lifted off the underlying cartilages.

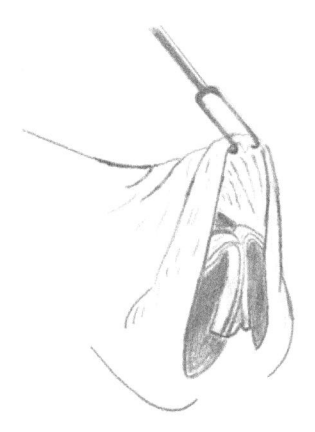

Then a hump of bone is removed from the bridge of the nose. This is done with a rasp or an osteotome (bone chisel).

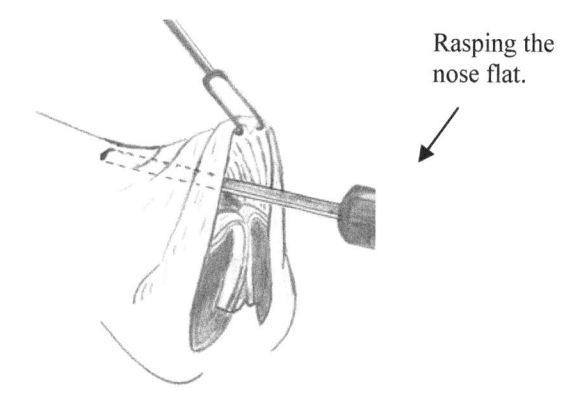

Rasping the nose flat.

This will flatten the nose, but it leaves a gap between the bones. The nose bones are therefore broken and pushed inwards to fill the gap left by removing the hump.

Everybody's Guide to Cosmetic Plastic Surgery

An osteotome and hammer are used to break the nasal bones.

Nasal bones

The nasal bones are then pushed inwards to fill the gap left from removing the hump.

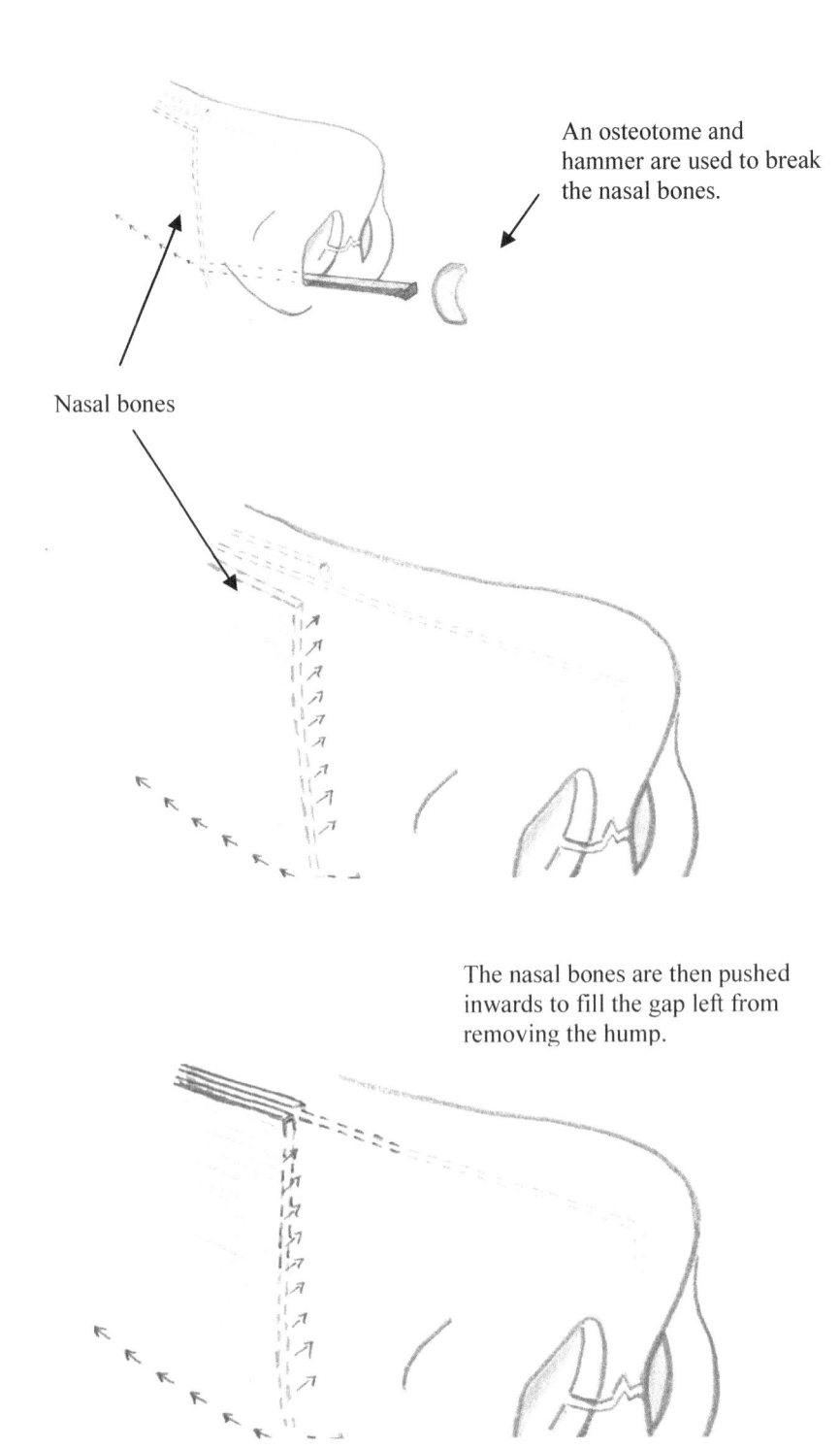

The cartilages in the tip of the nose are then made smaller and put into a better position. The whole operation takes about two hours.

Some nasal surgery involves the use of cartilage grafts. The cartilage is used to give extra support to noses which have an inadequate bridge or tip. The cartilage is taken from the septum of the nose or less commonly from an ear or a rib cartilage. These techniques are more commonly used for revision surgery.

What does nasal surgery involve?

The operation is done under a general anaesthetic. The patient will usually be admitted on the morning of surgery, be seen by the surgeon and anaesthetist and then be taken down to the operating theatre. The surgery takes about two hours. When they wake up they may have a "pack" in their nose. This is a piece of paraffin coated gauze which is inserted into the nose to help splint the bones and stop any bleeding. It will often be removed the next day. Patients may be uncomfortable at first and unable to breath through their nose. The nose will be swollen, and it will have a plaster of Paris splint over the top of it. This stays on for a week or two.

If all is well they should be able to go home the next day. It is usually possible to breath through the nose within a week. The surgery is often associated with a lot of bruising, especially around the eyes. This is normal, and reduces over the next two weeks. When the plaster is removed at a week the nose may still appear very swollen. The swelling will go down over the first month, but will not be back to normal for about six months.

What are the risks of nasal surgery?

Most rhinoplasties give good results with no complications. It can be a very satisfying procedure for both surgeon and patient, and many patients wish they had the courage to have it done sooner. However, there are some risks. Patients who have bleeding disorders, high blood pressure or heart disease should avoid this type of surgery. These conditions can cause excessive bleeding. It is rare, but if it happens it can require further surgery to stop it. More commonly the problem is one of aesthetics. Removing too much bone from the bridge can produce a "ski slope" nose, or conversely not removing enough can leave an uneven hump. The nose may be slightly deviated to one side after surgery, or the tip may be too small or too big. These are all correctable problems in the right hands, but they will all involve further surgery, often at the patients expense.

Rarer problems include blocked airways, perforations in the nasal septum and scar problems.

NASAL SURGERY (RHINOPLASTY)	
Cost	UK: £ 3,000 - £4,000 US: $5,000 - $6,000
Anaesthetic	General Anaesthetic
Hospital stay	Overnight
Recovery	14 days
Risks	Bleeding Prominent scar Asymmetry Residual Hump Excessive Hump removal Numbness of nasal tip Blocked nasal airway

9. Prominent Ear Correction

Prominent ears (bat ears) are a common anatomical variant, present in about 2% of the population. They are commonly corrected in childhood by surgery (an otoplasty), and there is some evidence that they can be corrected with splints within the first six weeks of life. However, many adults were never offered these opportunities as a child and wish to have their ears corrected in later life.

There are three anatomical variants that can make a patient's ears prominent.

> 1. The ear can be normal but at an abnormal angle to the head.

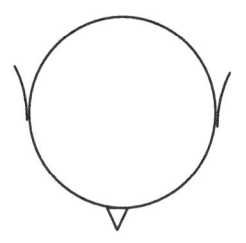

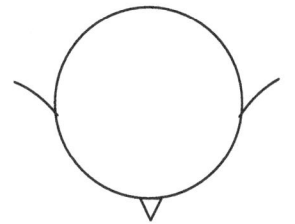

2. The cup of the ear (conchal fossa) may be too large.

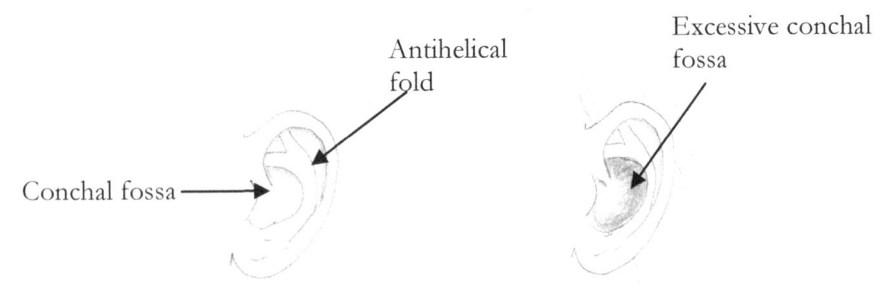

Conchal fossa →

Antihelical fold

Excessive conchal fossa

3. The fold on the outer part of the ear (antihelical fold) may not form properly

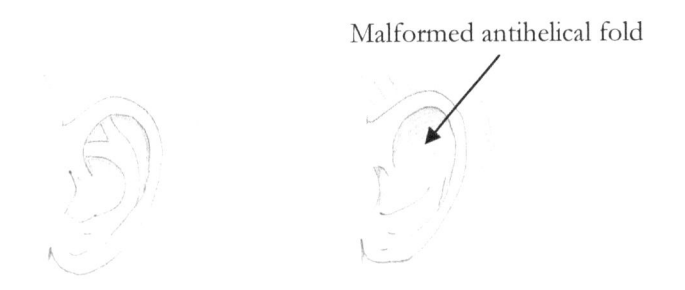

Malformed antihelical fold

How are prominent ears corrected?

The surgery involves making an incision behind the ear. The cartilage within the ear is then exposed and a combination of techniques are used to change the shape of the cartilage.

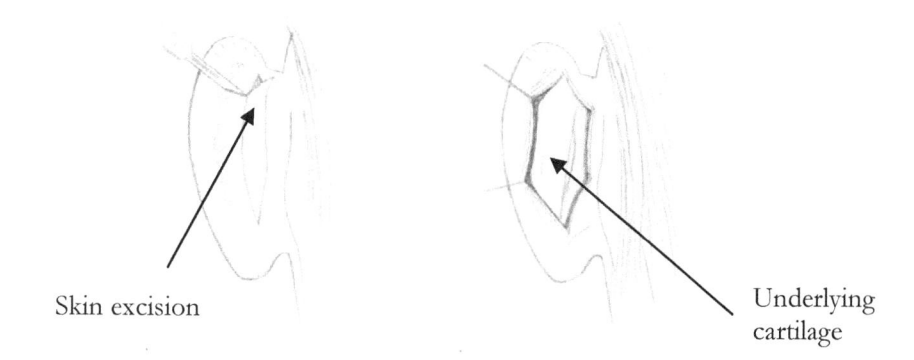

Skin excision

Underlying cartilage

This can be done by scoring the anterior surface of the cartilage with a scalpel. The weakened cartilage then folds back easily.

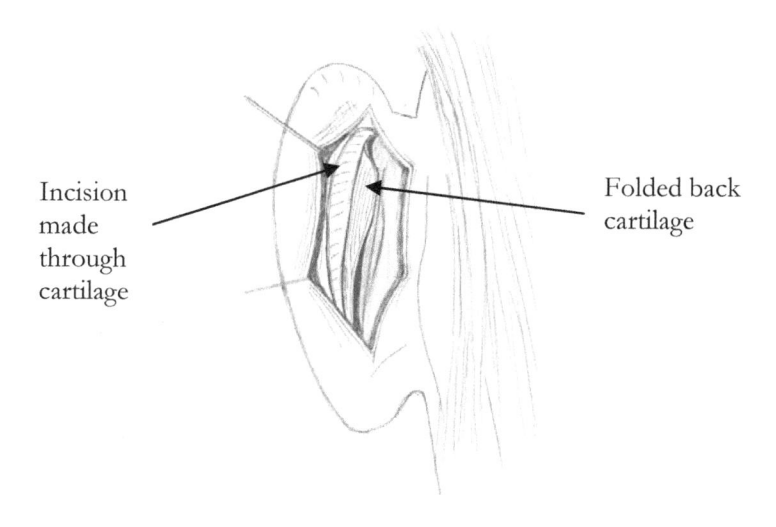

Incision made through cartilage

Folded back cartilage

Scoring the front surface of the cartilage

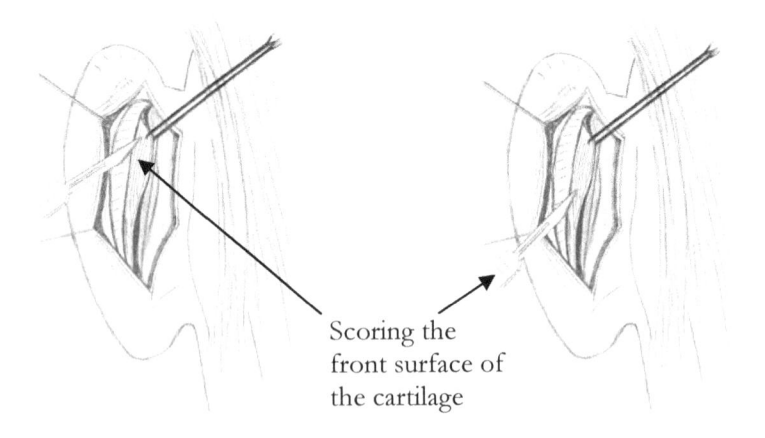

Alternatively some surgeons prefer to use buried sutures to change the shape of the cartilage or to hold it flat against the head.

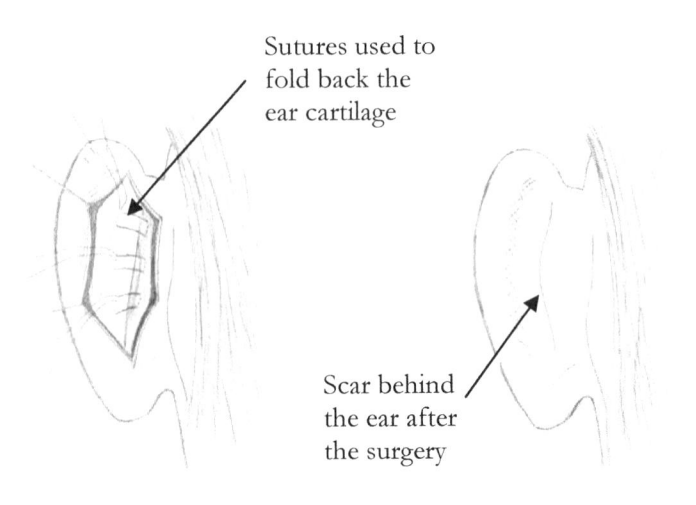

Sutures used to fold back the ear cartilage

Scar behind the ear after the surgery

If the cup of the ear is too large then a wedge of cartilage is removed from the cup to reduce its size. This can usually be done from behind the ear, but very occasionally a surgeon may make a small incision in the front of the ear to achieve this.

What does the surgery involve?

The operation is usually done under a general anaesthetic. It can be done under local anaesthetic but the injections in the ear are very painful. The operation takes about an hour. The surgeon and anaesthetist will see you on the morning of the surgery and then you will be taken down to theatre and put to sleep.

After the surgery a bandage is placed around the head. Most patients are able to go home the same day. The ears will usually be numb from local anaesthetic which is used to control any pain. The bandages are removed after several days, depending on the preferences of the surgeon. They can be removed in clinic. The sutures used to close the wound are often self-dissolving. If not any sutures will be removed after ten days. Patients are often advised to wear a head band at night for a further three months to protect the ears during sleep.

What are the risks of ear correction surgery?

The correction of prominent ears is one of the most commonly performed procedures. It is a safe and reliable operation. However, there are a number of complications which can occur.

A small percentage of patients (1 to 2%) will get a collection of blood forming within the ear in the first few days after surgery (a haematoma). This usually presents with excessive pain in the ear or sometimes blood discharging from the suture lines beneath the dressing. If suspected the bandages should be removed and the ears inspected. The ears will be swollen. It is important that this blood collection is drained. This will involve another operation, but it should not affect the end result of surgery. If the blood collection is not removed it will leave a very poor cosmetic result.

There is a small chance of a wound infection which can be treated with oral antibiotics. Very rarely this infection will involve the cartilage beneath the skin. If this happens then a long course of intravenous antibiotics may be needed. This may affect the shape of the ear. It is a serious but rare problem.

The scar from surgery is placed behind the ear and is not directly visible. However, sometimes this scar can become prominent (a hypertrophic scar). In a small number of individuals it can become very prominent (a keloid scar). This is a difficult problem to treat, often needing multiple steroid injections. It is more common in patients with dark skin, and adults who are susceptible will often know that they have a predilection to bad scars and should therefore avoid the surgery.

The surgeon will aim to place the ears into a normal anatomical position. However, they may be under-corrected (still slightly prominent) or over-corrected (too flat against the side of the head). There is often mild asymmetry after the surgery.

There is also a risk of the prominent ears recurring. This may require a repeat procedure to correct it.

The sensation in the ears may be reduced after surgery, though this often recovers fully. The ears may also suffer from cold intolerance and sometimes excessive sensitivity to touch. This will usually improve with time.

Prominent Ear Correction	
Cost	UK: £ 1,500 - £2,500 US: $2,000 - $4,000
Anaesthetic	General Anaesthetic
Hospital stay	Day Surgery
Recovery	1 – 2 weeks
Risks	Wound infection Haematoma Abnormal scar Asymmetry Cold intolerance Abnormal ear shape Ear hypersensitivity Recurrence Cartilage infection

10. Breast reduction surgery

Who benefits from a breast reduction?

Large breasts can be the foundation of several health problems. They can cause back pain and shoulder discomfort, skin maceration under the breasts and inability to exercise due to the weight of the breasts. These are all very valid reasons to request surgery. Patients may also be unhappy with the appearance of the breasts.

Many surgeons will measure the patient's weight and height before surgery. This gives a figure called the Body Mass Index (BMI). If it is over 30 then surgery can be risky, and patients may be asked to try to reduce their weight. The surgeon will do this for the patients safety, not because he or she does not wish to carry out the surgery.

If patients are over 55 or have a family history of breast cancer they should have a mammogram before the surgery. It is important that the surgeon perform a clinical examination for breast lumps in all patients prior to surgery.

How is a breast reduction done?

A breast reduction will reduce the size of the breasts by excising some of the breast tissue whilst preserving the nipple. There are several techniques for doing this. The main differences are the scars that will be left and the degree of disruption to nipple sensation. The two most common surgical techniques involve either a vertical scar or the inverted T scar. These are shown below. They both include a scar around the areola (the pigmented area around the nipple).

Vertical Scar Technique

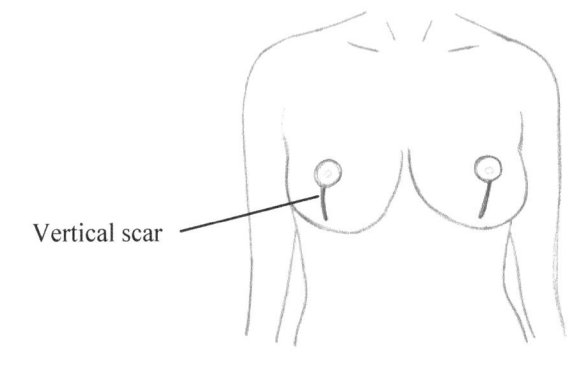

Breast Reduction

The vertical scar technique produces a scar around the areola and then a vertical scar below this. This technique was originally described by a French surgeon called Lassous and was popularised by Mme Lejour.

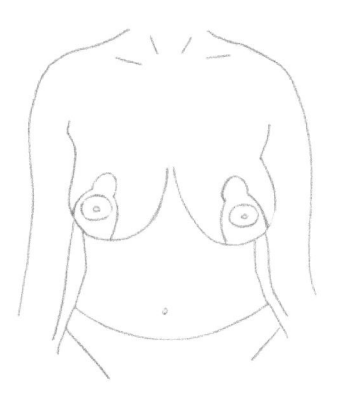

The surgeon will mark the breasts on the ward prior to surgery. During surgery the skin and breast tissue within the markings is excised. The nipple is moved upwards and then the breast tissue either side is sutured together to re-shape the breast.

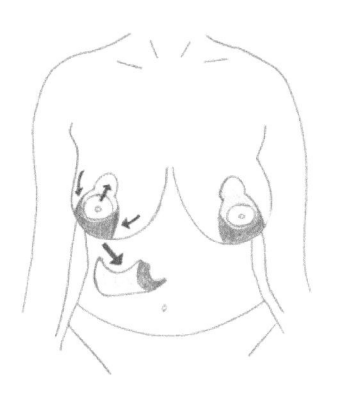

This produces a smaller scar than the inverted T technique, but it has two main drawbacks. Firstly, the shape of the breasts is often abnormal for the first couple of months.

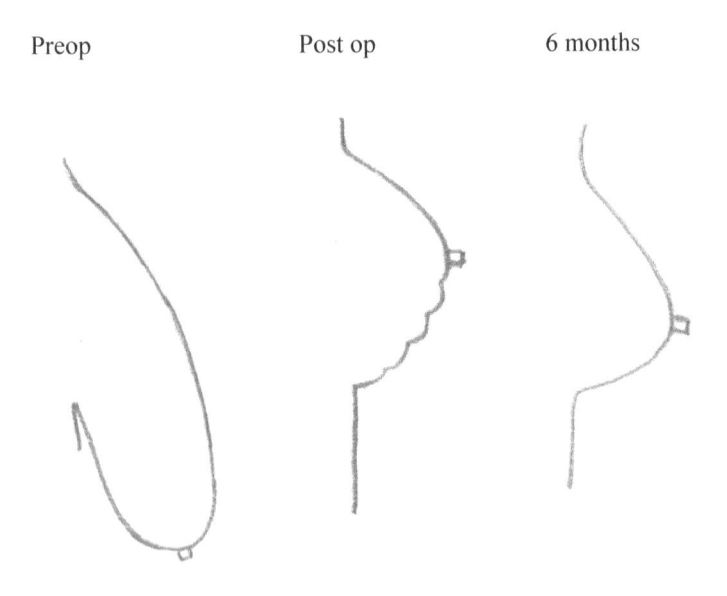

Preop   Post op   6 months

Secondly, fifteen to twenty percent of patient's will need revision surgery at the base of the scar.

Breast Reduction

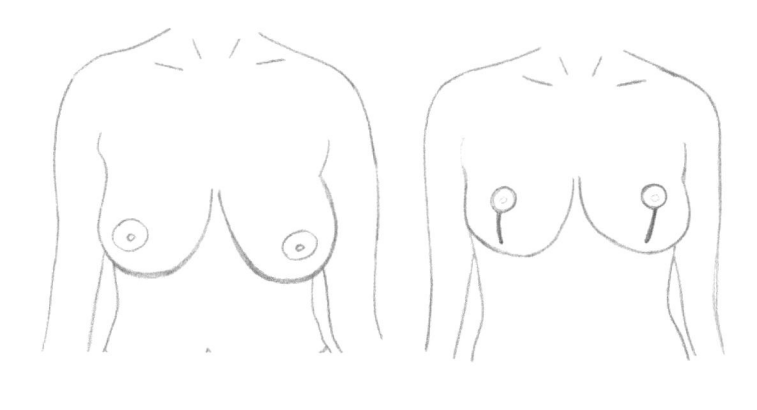

Pre-op   Post-op

Inverted T Scar Technique

The inverted T scar technique shown below produces a scar in the shape of an anchor. The scar lies around the areola and in a vertical line below it. There are also two horizontal limbs to the scar which run in the line of a bra under-wire (a line known as the inframammary fold).

Inverted T
scar

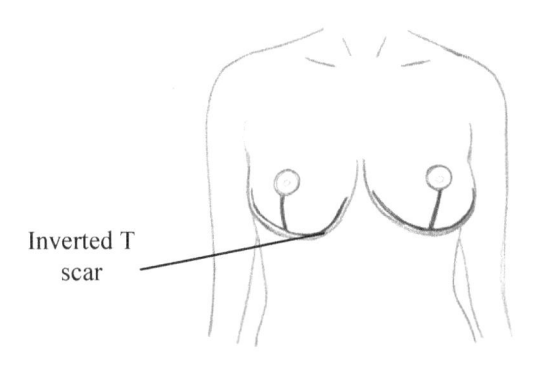

The surgeon will mark the breasts with a marker pen on the ward prior to surgery.

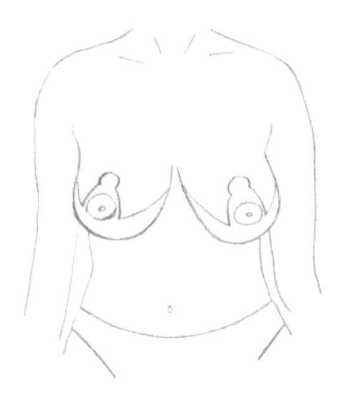

In the operating theatre the marked area of skin and breast tissue around the nipple is excised.

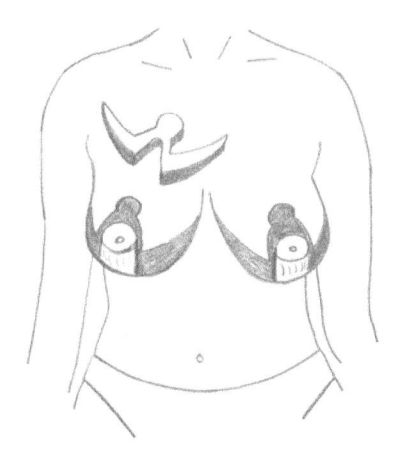

This excised tissue is discarded, and the nipple is moved upwards into the keyhole that has been created.

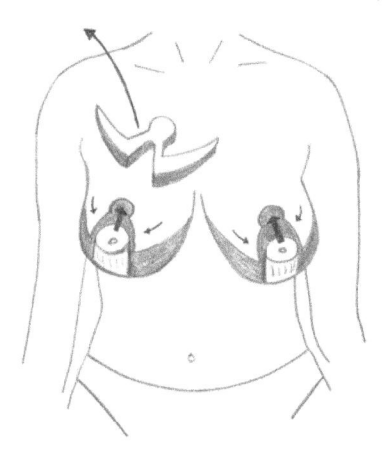

The surrounding skin is sutured to re-create the shape of the breast.

Pre-op   Post-op

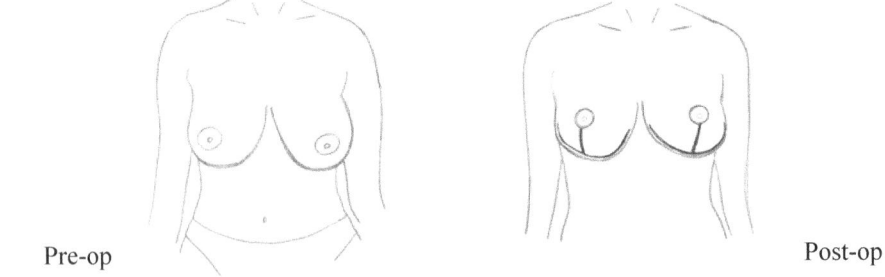

The inverted T technique (inferior pedicle) has a more extensive scar, but some surgeons feel that they have more control over the breast shape achieved. The main criticism of the technique is that the shape of the breast changes in time. The breasts are said to "bottom out" over time. The nipple starts to point upwards, with the bulk of the breast slumped below (shown below).

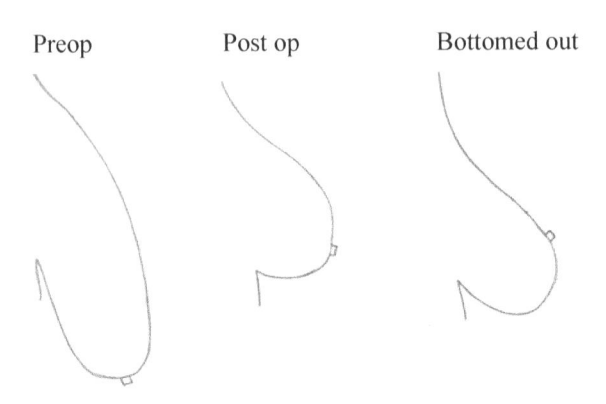

Preop   Post op   Bottomed out

A surgeon will often prefer to use one technique over the other. There is still some debate as to which technique is better. In reality, a surgeon will probably get the best results for you by using whichever technique he or she uses most commonly.

> **What do patients go through when they have a breast reduction?**

The operation is done under a general anaesthetic. Patients are usually admitted on the morning of surgery, seen by the surgeon and anaesthetist and then be taken down to the operating theatre. The surgery takes between one and three hours depending on how much tissue needs to be removed. When patients wake up they will have dressings over the wounds and may have a drain in each side. This is usually not a painful procedure but patients may need some simple analgesia. They will probably leave hospital the following day, after the drains have been removed. The breasts will be swollen at first and this will diminish over the next month or so. The recovery time from the procedure is variable, but patients will probably feel very tired for a couple of weeks and may need up to a month away from work. Patients with small children will need to have someone to help around the home as they will not be able to lift them or drive for two to three weeks. The wounds are usually healed within two weeks, but they are prone to breaking down in the lower part of the breast. This happens in about thirty percent of patients and can take six to eight weeks to heal. Occasionally a small skin graft is needed to speed this healing process up, but this is rare.

What are the risks of breast reduction surgery?

Most breast reductions can be a very satisfying procedure for both surgeon and patient. However, there are some risks, including some relatively common complications. I have already mentioned the length of time that may be needed for the wounds to heal. If you smoke you are very likely to have this problem.

The operation involves a general anaesthetic. Patients who are overweight at the time of surgery (i.e. have a high BMI) are at risk of having a deep vein thrombosis. This is a blood clot which can form in the veins of the leg. This blood clot can very occasionally travel from the leg to the lungs, causing a pulmonary embolus. This is a dangerous complication, although very rare. This is the reason why a surgeon may refuse to operate on some patients until they have lost some weight.

A small percentage of people having a breast reduction will develop a collection of blood in the wound within the first few days of surgery (a haematoma). This will require a second operation to remove the blood. It occurs in about five to ten percent of breast reduction operations.

Small areas of fat within the breast can become necrotic. This can cause a small collection that requires draining. This fat necrosis can also cause lumps to appear in the breast after a few months. They are harmless lumps but can cause anxiety. They can be distinguished from breast cancer lumps using mammography.

Once the wounds have healed they sometimes become red and lumpy. This happens in as many as twenty percent of patients. It can be helped by putting silicone gel or surgical tape on the wounds. This often settles after 6 to 8 months, but the scars may then look stretched and wide. Sometimes a revision procedure is needed to remove excess skin left at the end of the scars (dog ears).

The nipple can also be affected by the surgery. Often its sensation will be reduced after the surgery. However, seventy percent of patients will still have reasonable sensation. Sometimes the blood supply to the nipples is disrupted by the operation. The nipple can suffer partial or complete necrosis. This is not common, occurring in less than one percent of patients. Nipples can be reconstructed, but this will require further surgery. Women who plan to have children in the future need to consider that breast reduction surgery will reduce their chances of breast feeding. Studies have shown that about seventy percent of women who have had a breast reduction are able to breast feed, with a slight variation depending on the technique used. We must remember that not all women would be able to breast feed anyway.

Most women who have breast reduction surgery are delighted with the result. It is important to tell the surgeon what you would like to achieve as there is always a risk of removing not enough breast tissue or too much. Most women have asymmetrical breasts, and this may still be the case after surgery. Any asymmetry of the nipples may also be accentuated by the surgery.

Women who have breast reduction surgery get a fantastic improvement in symptoms such as back and shoulder pain and most experience a significant improvement in appearance and self-confidence.

BREAST REDUCTION SURGERY	
Cost	UK: £4,000 - £6,000 US: $5,000 - $6,000
Anaesthetic	General Anaesthetic
Hospital stay	1 - 2 days
Recovery	2 - 4 weeks
Risks	Wound infection Prominent scars Haematoma Fat necrosis Breast asymmetry Breasts too small Breasts too large Nipple numbness Nipple asymmetry Nipple loss Inability to breast feed

11. Breast Lift Surgery (Mastopexy)

Who benefits from a breast lift?

Breasts undergo several changes throughout life. They increase in size at puberty. During pregnancy there is a further increase in size due to hypertrophy (increase in size and number) of the breast glands which produce milk. This resolves when breast feeding ceases, with a reduction in overall breast size. This fluctuation in size recurs with subsequent pregnancies.

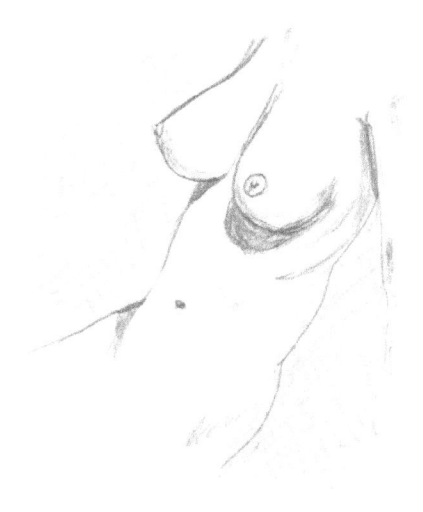

The supporting structures within the breast become lax with increasing age. This is exacerbated by the fluctuations in breast weight and hormone levels. The position of the breasts changes with time and they lie lower on the chest wall. Also the position of the nipple will change with time. In the young breast the nipple lies above the lower pole of the breast, with age the nipple will fall below the lowest part of the breast. Women often complain that their nipples "point to the floor".

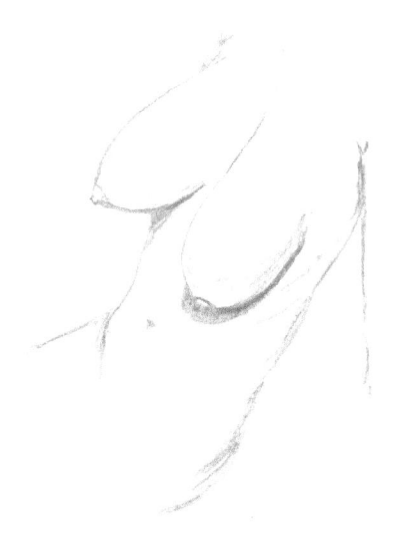

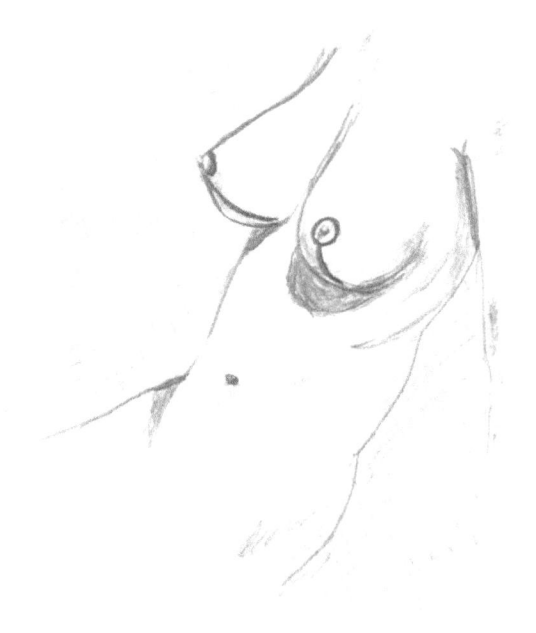

A breast lift or mastopexy is designed to correct this problem. The procedure will also help to correct breast shape in women who have asymmetric breast shape or nipple position. It can be combined with a breast augmentation. It is very important that patients understand exactly what the operation involves and the likely scars before deciding to have a breast lift. The scars are extensive for what may be a relatively minor improvement in shape. Patients planning to have more children should postpone breast lift surgery. Pregnancy is likely to stretch the breasts again and offset the results of the procedure.

Patients over 55 or anyone with a family history of breast cancer should have a mammogram before the surgery. It is important that the surgeon perform a clinical examination for breast lumps in all patients.

What does breast lift surgery involve?

A breast lift will improve the shape of the breasts by excising some of the excess skin and repositioning the nipple. There are several techniques for doing this. The main differences are the scars produced and the degree of disruption to nipple sensation.

The extent of the scar often depends on the distance the nipple needs to be moved. If the nipple does not need to move very far, then a scar around the areola may suffice. This is called a peri-areola mastopexy.

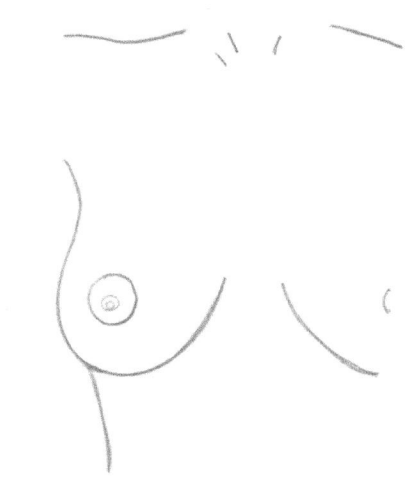

Peri-areola mastopexy – an incision is made around the nipple

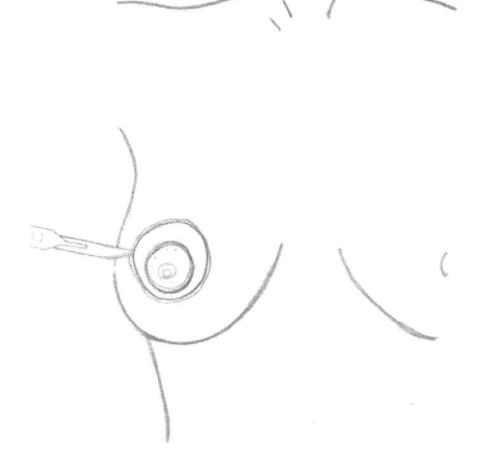

Everybody's Guide to Cosmetic Plastic Surgery

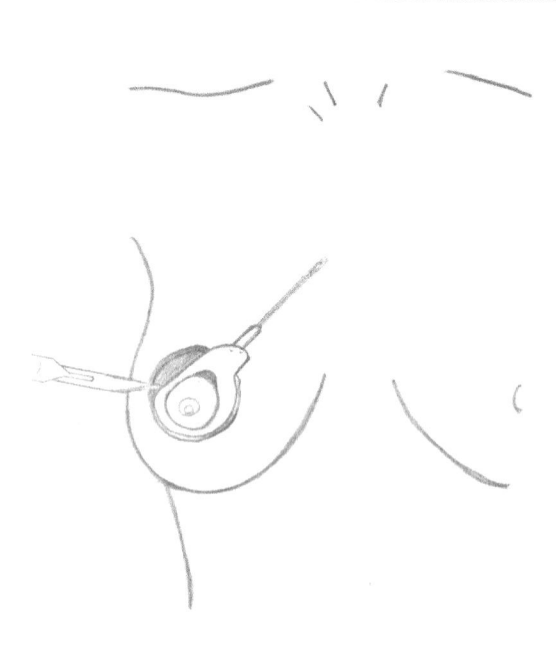

The skin around the nipple is excised.

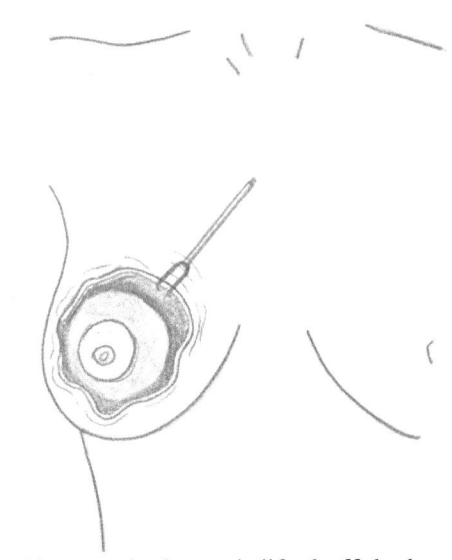

The skin over the breast is lifted off the breast tissue.

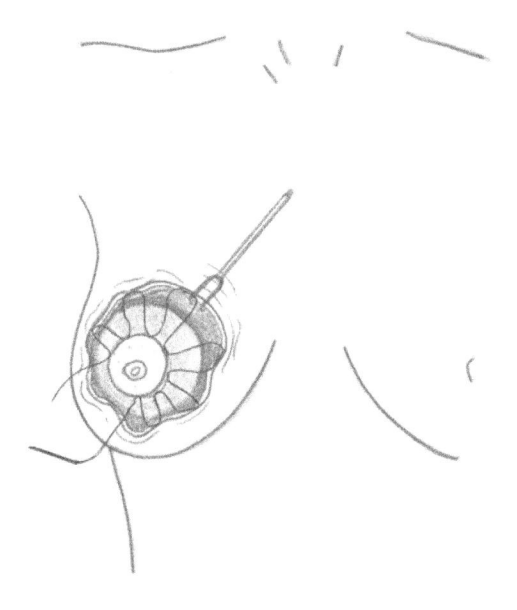

A 'purse-string' suture is passed around the nipple and onto the skin over the breast to pull it together. This raises the nipple and tightens the breast skin.

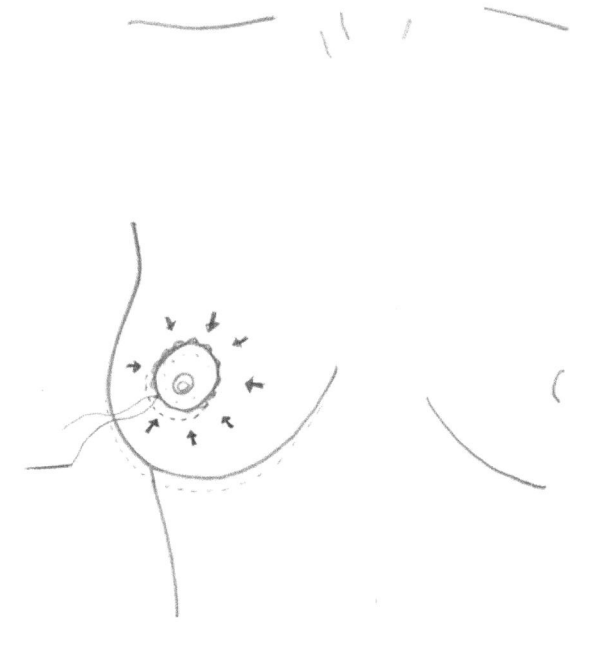

If the nipple needs to be moved further then a peri-areola scar with a vertical scar below it will be needed.

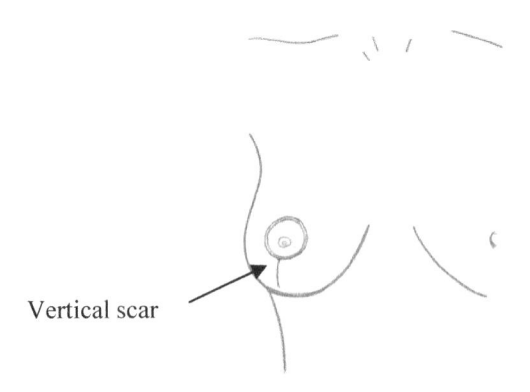

Vertical scar

Breasts which are very lax with excess poor quality skin (needing a very large change in nipple position) are difficult to correct. They can only be improved with surgery that produces a peri-areola and an inverted T scar as shown below.

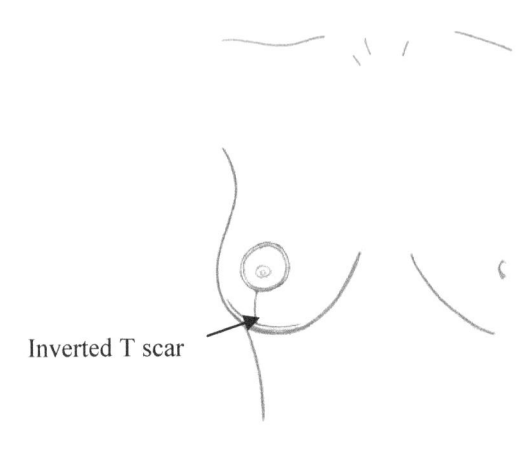

Inverted T scar

Sometimes the surgeon may decide that the shape of the breast can best be improved by augmenting the size of the breasts with an implant. The extra volume in the breast will improve the position of the nipples and improve any skin laxity. Occasionally a combination of augmentation and a breast lift is needed. This can be done in one stage or more safely in two separate operations. Breast augmentation is discussed in the next chapter.

What does a breast lift involve for the patient?

The operation is done under a general anaesthetic. Patients are usually admitted the morning of surgery, are seen by the surgeon and anaesthetist and are then taken down to theatre. The surgery takes between one and two hours. When patients wake up they will have dressings over the wounds and may have a drain in each side. This is usually not a painful procedure but patients often need some simple analgesia. Most people leave hospital the following day, after the drains have been removed. The breasts will be swollen at first and this will diminish over the next month or so. The recovery time from the procedure is variable. Patients will need a couple of weeks off work. If they have small children they will need to have someone to help around the home as they will not be able to lift them or drive for two to three weeks. The wounds are usually healed within two weeks and any sutures will be removed at this time.

What are the risks of having a breast lift?

A small percentage of people having a breast lift will develop a collection of blood in the wound within the first few days of surgery (a haematoma). This will require a second operation to remove the blood. It occurs in about five percent of breast lift procedures.

Once the wounds have healed they sometimes become red and raised. This happens in as many as thirty percent of patients. It can be helped by putting silicone gel or surgical tape on the wounds. This often settles after 6 to 8 months.

The nipples can also be affected by the surgery. The sensation can be reduced, or they can become hyper-sensitive. The blood supply to the nipples can also be reduced by the operation. The nipple can suffer partial or complete necrosis.

Women who plan to have children in the future need to consider that breast lift surgery can reduce their chances of breast feeding. Likewise, pregnancy and breast feeding will reverse the improvements created by surgery.

BREAST LIFT SURGERY (MASTOPEXY)	
Cost	UK: £ 4,000 - £6,000 US: $5,000 - $6,000
Anaesthetic	General Anaesthetic
Hospital stay	1 - 2 days
Recovery	2 - 4 weeks
Risks	Haematoma Wound infection Prominent scars Breast asymmetry Nipple numbness Nipple asymmetry Nipple loss Inability to breast feed

12. Breast Augmentation Surgery

Breast augmentation is one of the most controversial operations in the history of plastic surgery. Implants have developed significantly over the last few decades. There are now at least four generations of silicone implant, each differing from the former.

Who benefits from breast augmentation surgery?

Anyone who thinks their breasts are too small may benefit from breast implants.

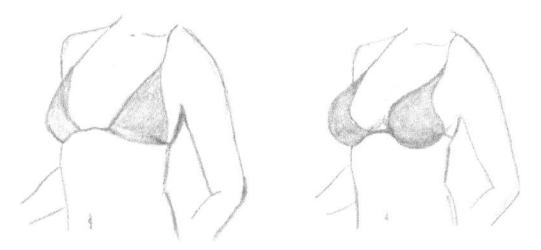

Women with asymmetric breasts can be treated by putting implants into each breast which are slightly different sizes. A larger implant is inserted on the side of the smaller breast.

Types of Breast Implant

Modern breast implants are of two main types, silicone or saline. Both have an outer solid silicone shell, but one type is filled with silicone, the other with saline. Soya bean and Hydrogel implants are no longer licensed for use in the UK.

The silicone filled implants can likewise be divided into two types, those filled with a fluid type of silicone, or those filled with a gel form of silicone (cohesive gel silicone implants). The decision to use saline or silicone is up to individual patients. Saline probably has a better safety profile, but they are often poor mimics of breast tissue. If they rupture they will deflate immediately, leaving asymmetric breasts. Silicone implants have a more natural feel and the cohesive gel implants will not leak silicone into the surrounding tissue if they rupture.

Implant Shape

The shape of an implant can be either round (above) or anatomical (below).

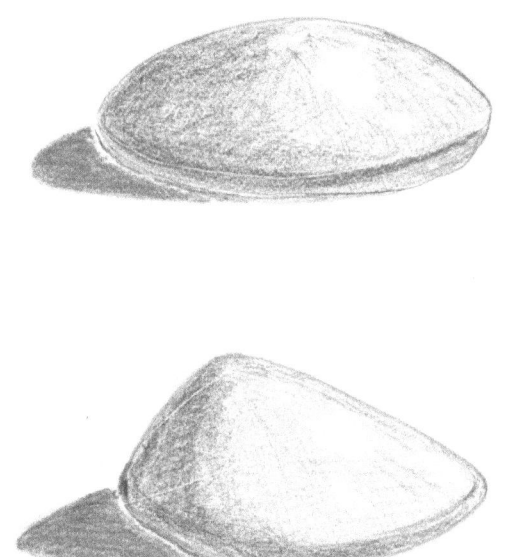

Anatomical implants are also sometimes called contoured implants. They are shaped like a tear drop to better mimic the shape of the breast. The results are often similar with both types of implant, though anatomical implants may look more natural in thin women. Unfortunately, they can occasionally rotate after insertion which may cause problems.

Implant Shell

The shell of all implants is made from solid silicone. This silicone shell may be either smooth or textured. Most surgeons now believe that textured surfaces reduce the rate of capsular contraction.

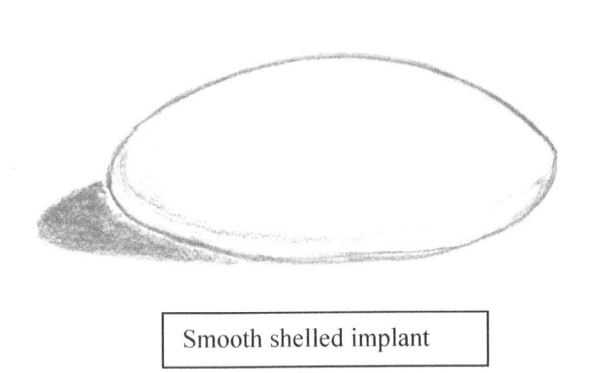

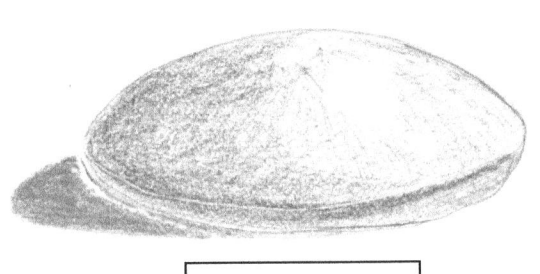

Smooth shelled implant

Textured implant

Implant Size

Implant size is measured in cubic centimetres (cc) or millilitres (ml). Implants of about 250 cc will increase the breasts by one bra size. This is only a very rough guide to choosing an implant. A better estimate of the implant size needed can be made by filling a latex glove with water or rice. This is then placed over the breast in a sports bra. The volume of water is then adjusted to the desired size and the volume of water measured.

Implants also have different diameters and projection. The ideal implant will be chosen by your surgeon with your guidance. The final result also depends on other factors. These include the shape and symmetry of the rib cage, the size and shape of the breast and the quality of the skin.

The Silicone Debate

Silicone-gel breast implants first went on the market in 1962. Thirty years later, they were banned in the United States amid concerns about their safety. There has since been heated debate over the safety of silicone. It was linked to a syndrome known as Human Adjuvant Disease (with similarities to forms of arthritis). However, several large studies have now shown that there is probably no such entity, and that anecdotal reports of a link between silicone and rheumatoid like illnesses was due to the natural occurrence of these problems in the 2 million American women who had already had breast implants. A recent report by the Institute of Medicine in America and by the Independent Review Group in the UK has highlighted that the most significant problems with silicone breast implants are local complications, namely capsular contracture and implant rupture. Saline filled implants are also affected by these two complications.

In America the FDA has now approved the following implants:

- "In May 2000, Mentor and Allergan (formerly Inamed) received approval for saline-filled breast implants. These implants were approved for breast augmentation in women 18 years or older and for breast reconstruction in women of any age."
- "In November 2006, Allergan and Mentor received approval for their silicone gel-filled breast implants. These implants were approved for breast augmentation in women 22 years or older and for breast reconstruction in women of any age."

All other breast implants used in America can only be used as part of a clinical trial.

In the UK breast implants are under the regulatory authority of the Medicines and Healthcare products Regulatory Agency (MHRA), an executive agency of the Department of Health. There are no restrictions on the sale or use of CE-marked silicone gel-filled breast implants.

Implants and Breast Cancer

Currently there is no evidence of a link between breast implants and breast cancer. A clinical examination to exclude breast lumps is a mandatory part of the pre-operative assessment for all patients. Patients over 55 should have pre-operative mammography to exclude suspicious breast lesions.

There is still some debate regarding breast cancer detection in women with implants. The breast tissue is displaced by the implants, making mammography difficult. Routine screening in older patients requires special mammography views (Ekland views) in patients with implants, but recent studies have shown that breast cancer detection is not delayed in these patients.

Incisions for Breast Implants

There are four incisions that can be used to place the implant beneath the breast. These are listed in order of popularity:

- Infra-mammary – beneath the breast
- Peri-areola – around the nipple
- Axilla – through the armpit
- Umbilical – through the belly button

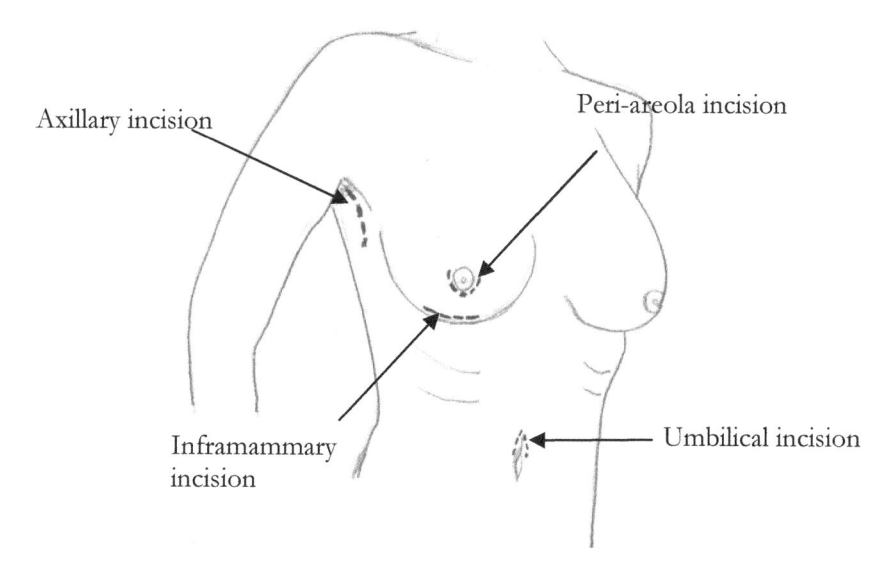

Axillary incision

Peri-areola incision

Inframammary incision

Umbilical incision

The surgeon will place the implant either under the breast tissue or under the chest wall muscle.

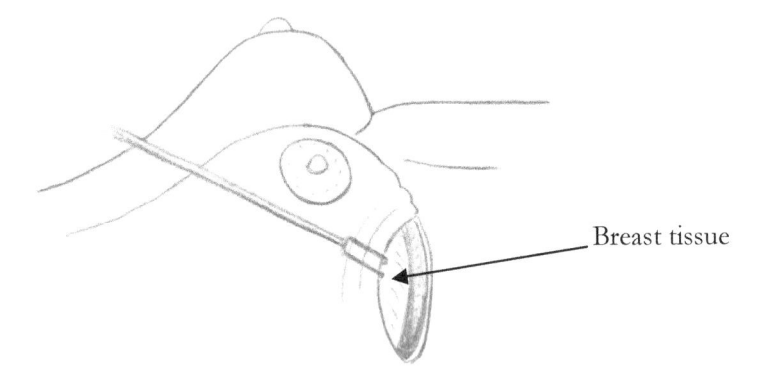

Everybody's Guide to Cosmetic Plastic Surgery

Breast tissue

Sub-mammary Implant Placement

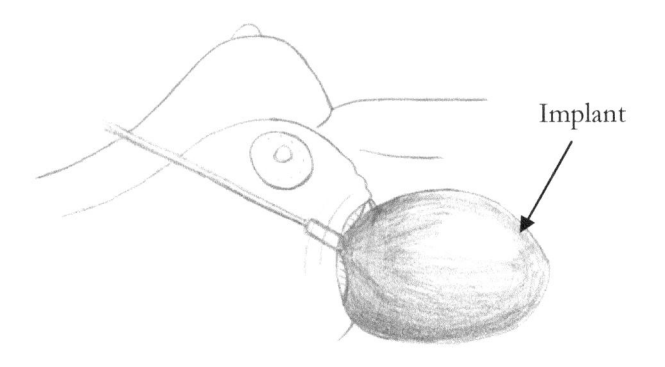

Implant

Sub-mammary Implant Placement

Breast tissue
Implant

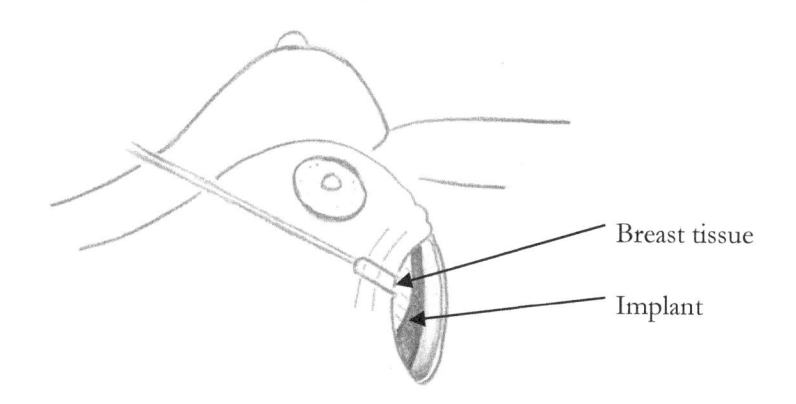

There is some evidence that implants placed beneath the muscle will have a lower rate of capsule formation. Sub-muscular positioning (under the muscle and breast) will also reduce the risk of the implant edges showing in very thin patients. The criticism of sub-muscular placement is that sometimes the implants move with contraction of the muscle. This can be problematic in athletic women. They can also produce a "double bubble" appearance with the breast sitting as a separately contoured mound over the implant.

The sub-mammary implant position (under the breast tissue) allows more control of breast shape, especially when a contoured implant is used. The operation is also slightly shorter and the recovery shorter.

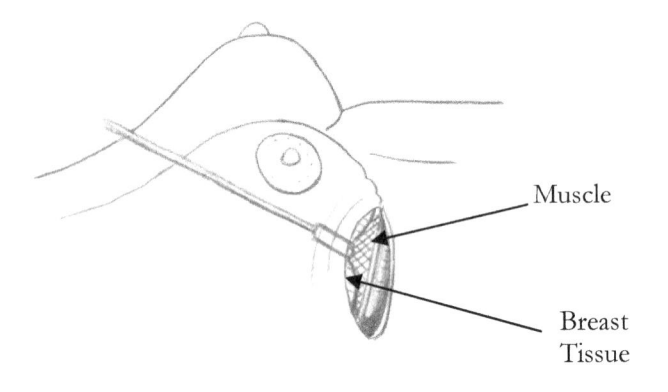

Sub-muscular Implant Placement

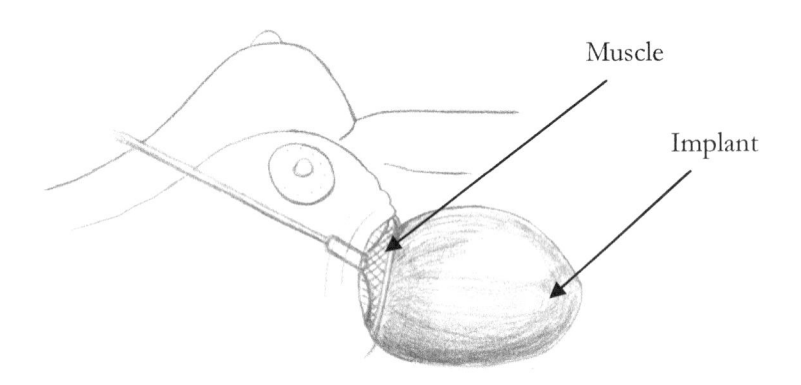

144

What does breast augmentation involve for the patient?

The operation is done under a general anaesthetic. Patients are usually admitted on the morning of surgery, are seen by the surgeon and anaesthetist and are then taken down to the operating theatre. The operation takes between one and two hours.

When the patient wakes up they will have dressings over the wounds and may have a drain in each side. They will probably leave hospital the following day, after the drains have been removed. The breasts may be swollen at first and will reduce in size over the next week or two. Most people will not be able to drive or do any heavy lifting for a couple of weeks.

What are the risks of breast augmentation surgery?

A small percentage of women having a breast augmentation will develop a collection of blood in the wound within the first few days of surgery (a haematoma). This will require a second operation to remove the blood. It occurs in about one to five percent of breast augmentation procedures.

Wound infection occurs in one to two percent of patients. It presents itself as a red and painful wound. This is usually only superficial, but rarely the implant can become infected. This will then have to be removed and can only be replaced after a settling down period of several months.

Scars can sometimes become red and raised. This can be helped by putting silicone gel or surgical tape on the wounds. This often settles after 6 to 8 months.

The nipples can also be affected by the surgery. Often the sensation will be reduced, but sometimes they may become hypersensitive. Women who plan to have children in the future need to consider that breast augmentation surgery may reduce their chances of breast feeding.

Most people have asymmetrical breasts, and this may still be the case after surgery. Any asymmetry of the nipples may also be accentuated by the surgery.

When the implants are inserted they can sometimes develop wrinkles and folds. These may be palpable in thin patients. The edge of the implant may also be visible. If this does not worry the patient it can be left. However, it is often not tolerated by patients and may require the implants to be exchanged.

Capsular contracture remains one of the most common complications of breast augmentation surgery. Thick scar tissue forms around the implant which contracts, changing the shape of the implant. The implant becomes spherical. It displaces the overlying breast tissue and the breast becomes firm, painful and looks unnatural. If it becomes symptomatic the only treatment is to remove the implant with or without the capsule and replace it.

The frequency of capsular contracture is thought to be lowest when using textured implants which are placed in a sub-muscular position. The exact incidence is unknown. Some studies have shown that over seventy percent of implants will develop a capsular contracture within 10 years. Many of these studies used older generation implants and techniques, and may not reflect current trends. More recent studies have shown rates of capsular contracture of about ten to fifteen percent.

Implant rupture is often difficult to detect. Many women have ruptured implants which are completely asymptomatic. Modern implants contain a cohesive gel which will not leak even if the outer shell ruptures. The exact rates of implant rupture are not known. Studies looking at older implants which needed removal showed rates as high as seventy percent. However, modern implants seem to have a rupture rate closer to ten percent over five years.

Most surgeons agree that women who decide to have implants will need further surgery at some stage in the future. This may be for a variety of reasons, but the augments will need lifelong maintenance and patients must consider both the physical, psychological and financial implications of this prior to embarking on breast augmentation surgery.

Despite these problems women who have had breast implants report that their self-esteem is considerably enhanced. They report that they feel more attractive, less self-conscious and more feminine.

BREAST AUGMENTATION	
Cost	UK: £ 4,000 - £5,000 US: $6,000 - $5,000
Anaesthetic	**General Anaesthetic**
Hospital stay	**1 - 2 days**
Recovery	**2 - 3 weeks**
Risks	**Wound infection** Wound breakdown **Haematoma** Seroma **Prominent scars** Breast pain **Breast asymmetry** Nipple asymmetry Nipple numbness Nipple hypersensitivity Implant infection

Risks (cont)	**Implant extrusion** **Implant rupture** **Implant displacement** **Implant rippling/ wrinkling** **Capsule formation** **Inability to breast feed** **Breast screening issues** **Silicone issues**

13. Tummy Tuck (Abdominoplasty)

Who benefits from a tummy tuck?

The abdomen (or tummy as it is often called) is made up of muscle and fat. The muscles form a cylinder around the abdominal contents, keeping them from bulging out. The fat surrounds this layer of muscle. It is there to keep us warm and to act as a food store. With age and pregnancy the muscles become lax, and we often put on extra fat. The skin over the abdomen can also become stretched, producing "stretch marks" or "striae". A tummy tuck (or abdominoplasty) is an operation which aims to correct these problems.

The best way to improve the shape of your waist is through diet and exercise. This will reduce the fat around the muscle and the increased muscle tone will help prevent the abdominal contents from bulging out.

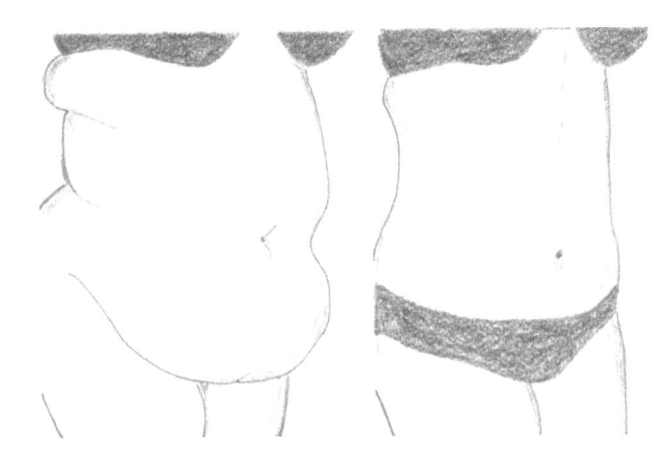

Pre- and Post-op abdominoplasty.

Men differ from women in several ways. Obviously they don't go through the "stretching" effect of pregnancy, but also the distribution of fat is very different. Men tend to gain fat within the abdomen rather than outside the muscle layer. This type of weight gain responds to dieting but cannot be easily removed with an abdominoplasty.

Sometimes diet and exercise will improve one's appearance only so much. Many women who have eaten a healthy diet and exercised regularly still have a small area of excess fat and skin around and below the umbilical region (belly button). This problem is often associated with stretch marks. This group of patients will get the best results from an abdominoplasty.

Patients who are still gaining weight are certainly not good candidates for an abdominoplasty. They will be disappointed as they continue to gain weight after the operation despite having the scars of surgery.

The risks associated with surgery are significantly increased in patients who smoke and have a high BMI (see page 72). There is no upper age limit for this type of surgery, but other medical problems such as heart disease, hypertension, diabetes or a previous deep vein thrombosis will increase the risk of anaesthetic complications. An abdominoplasty is a relatively major procedure.

How is an abdominoplasty done?

An abdominoplasty involves making an incision across the lower part of the abdomen and removing a wedge of skin and fat.

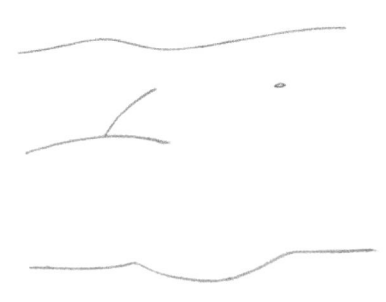

Abdominoplasty skin markings

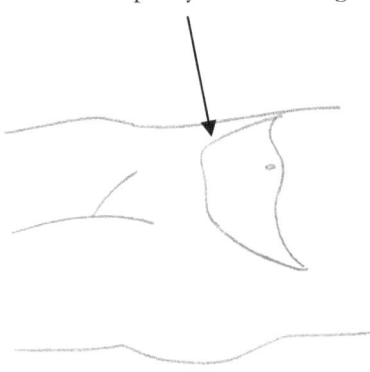

Excision of excess skin

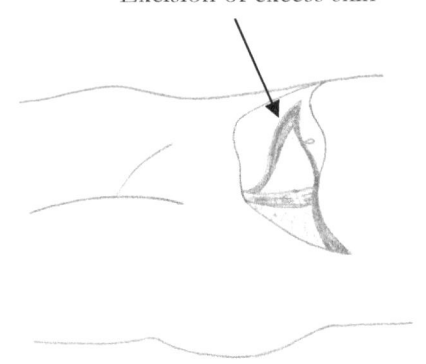

Abdominoplasty

                                                               Rectus muscles

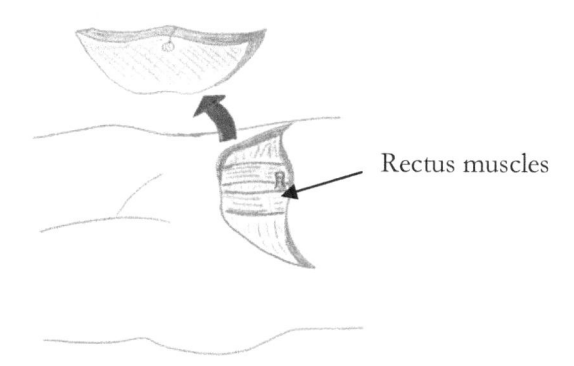

If the abdominal muscles are very lax (called a divarification of the rectus muscles) the surgeon may be able to tighten them.

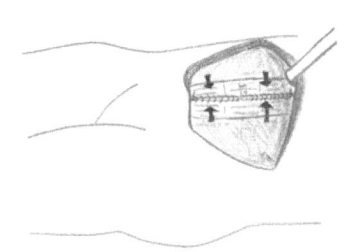

Tightening of the rectus muscles.

When this has been done the skin edges are sewn back together, but this buries the umbilicus (tummy button). Therefore the umbilicus has to be moved back up to the skin surface. This will produce a scar around it.

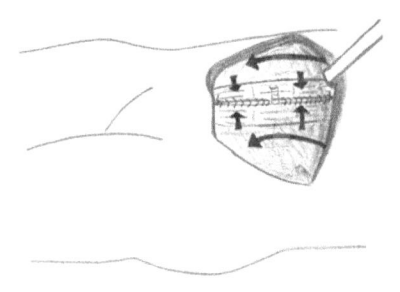

Closure of the skin flap.

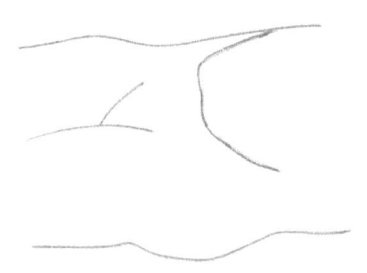

Retrieval of the umbilicus.

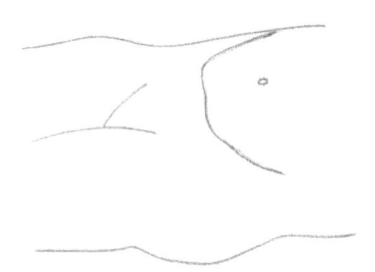

The final scar is usually at the level of the bikini. Patients can choose the position of the scar depending on the type of bikini they wear. It can be made straight across the tummy or in a more V shape if they prefer to wear hipster bikinis.

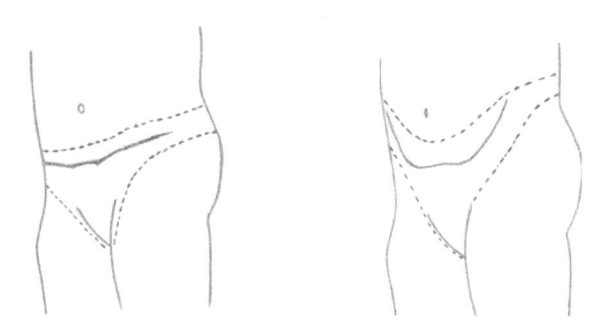

What does an abdominoplasty involve?

The operation is done under a general anaesthetic (you will be asleep). Patients are admitted on the morning of surgery, are seen by the surgeon and anaesthetist and are then taken down to the operating theatre. The surgery takes about two hours depending on how much tissue needs to be removed. Patients will have dressings over the wounds and may have a drain in each side. When they wake up they will have some pillows under their knees to keep their legs slightly flexed. This takes any tension off the wound on the abdomen. It may be slightly painful, but they will have some analgesia, or sometimes even an epidural.

The drains will be removed when they stop filling with fluid, which often takes a couple of days. Patients should be up and about the next day. They will probably be in hospital for two or three days. The abdomen will be swollen at first and this will diminish over the next month or so.

The recovery time from the procedure is variable, but most people will probably feel very tired for a couple of weeks and may need up to a month away from work. If they have small children they will need to have someone to help around the home as they will not be able to lift them or drive for two to three weeks. The wounds are usually healed within two weeks, and any sutures will be removed in the outpatient clinic at this time.

What are the risks of an abdominoplasty?

The operation involves a general anaesthetic. Patients who are overweight at the time of surgery (have a high BMI) will be at risk of having a chest infection or developing a deep vein thrombosis. This is a blood clot which can form in the veins of the leg. This blood clot can very occasionally travel from the leg to the lungs, causing a pulmonary embolus. This is a dangerous complication, although very rare. It is the reason why a surgeon may refuse to operate on patients till they have lost some weight. The risks are greatest in people who smoke and those who are on the oral contraceptive pill.

A small percentage of people having a tummy tuck will develop a collection of blood in the wound within the first few days of surgery (a haematoma). This will require a second operation to remove the blood. It occurs in about five to ten percent of people having a tummy tuck. Rarely this can cause some skin around the wound to become necrotic. If this happens it will need to be removed and may need a small skin graft. Fortunately this is very rare.

A similar problem can occur slightly later in the recovery period when a collection of fluid called serum can develop under the skin. This can often be removed with a needle and syringe, but the process may need to be repeated.

Once the wounds have healed they sometimes become red and raised. This happens in as many as twenty percent of patients. It can be helped by putting silicone gel or surgical tape on the wounds. This often settles after 6 to 8 months, but the scars may then look stretched and wide. The scar around the belly button can also be affected.

The skin of the abdomen may be numb after the surgery. This is due to nerves being cut or stretched during the operation. There will be some recovery of sensation over the first year or so, but there may always be some abnormal sesation.

Rarely the blood supply to the belly button (umbilicus) gets cut off by the surgery. This will then become necrotic and will need to be removed. It can be reconstructed at a later date, but this will involve more surgery. When performing the abdominoplasty the surgeon will try his best to remove the same amount of tissue from either side. However, sometimes there is some residual asymmetry after the operation. This may be asymmetry of the scar, of the fat or of the belly button.

The scar from an abdominoplasty will often extend round the flanks. At the ends of the scar "dog ears" of skin sometimes remain. These often need to be excised in a second procedure.

Despite all these potential problems the majority of women are very happy with the results. It gives them a massive boost in self esteem and confidence and is often the catalyst to a healthier and happier lifestyle.

ABDOMINOPLASTY (TUMMY TUCK)	
Cost	UK: £ 4,000 - £6,000 US: $6,000 - $8,000
Anaesthetic	General Anaesthetic
Hospital stay	2 - 5 days
Recovery	3 - 4 weeks
Risks	**Wound infection** **Wound breakdown** **Prominent scars** **Bleeding** **Asymmetry** **Numbness** **Umbilical asymmetry** **Umbilical loss**

14. Liposuction

Who benefits from Liposuction?

Liposuction can be used to remove excess fat. Unfortunately, it is no substitute for exercise and a healthy diet. The best candidates for liposuction are people who have a steady weight, but have small areas of fat which they are unable to get rid of by dieting and exercise. Patients who continue to eat excessively after liposuction soon regain their preoperative body shape.

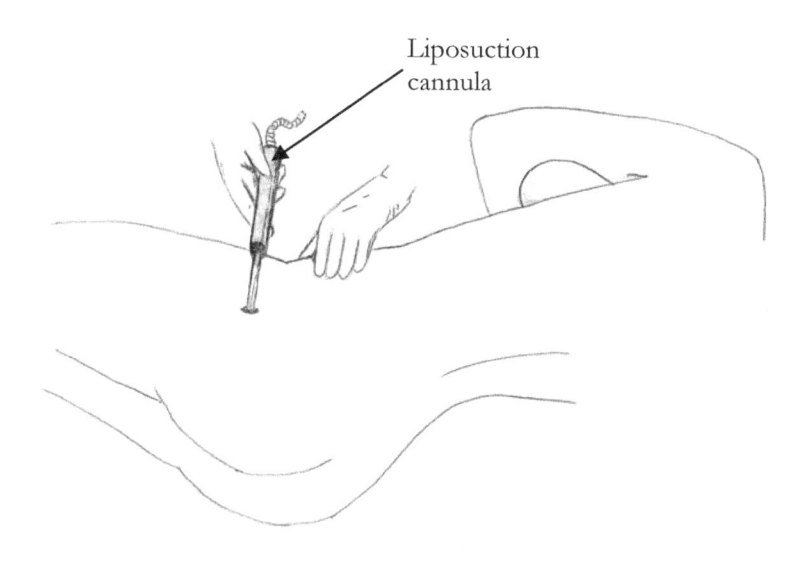

Liposuction cannula

Liposuction is not good at removing cellulite or stretch marks.

How is liposuction done?

Liposuction involves the removal of fat using a long thin cannula which is attached to a suction tube. The cannula is inserted through a very small incision made in the skin and then passed backwards and forwards into the area where fat needs to be removed.

Liposuction can be performed on many parts of the body. Some areas respond much better than others. The abdomen, thighs and buttocks are relatively easy to treat. Arms and legs, however, respond less well to treatment. There is a limit to how much surgery can be done in one go. Several operations may be needed to treat different areas if a lot of fat needs to be removed.

What does liposuction involve?

The operation is done under a general anaesthetic. Patients are admitted on the morning of surgery, are seen by the surgeon and anaesthetist and then taken down to the operating theatre. When they wake up they will have a few small incisions over the areas treated, each less than one centimetre long. They may have a stitch in them, or just a small dressing over the top. Many surgeons put their patients straight into a pressure garment, which is a very tight fitting elastic body suit which helps to compress the areas treated. This reduces post operative swelling. Most patients go home the next day, but the pressure garments are best worn for up to three months. Any sutures will be removed within the next two weeks. Patients will be relatively sore after the surgery, and may take a couple of weeks before returning to work.

What are the risks of liposuction?

Liposuction is a relatively safe procedure. In the hands of an experienced surgeon it can give very good results. There are some problems which are commonly seen, and some more rarely. The most dangerous complication which all surgeons fear is the patient developing a deep vein thrombosis. Many patients undergoing liposuction will have a high Body Mass Index (BMI see page 72) and are more susceptible to developing a venous thrombosis. This is still rare. If a DVT does occur it can pass through the bloodstream into the lungs causing serious illness and very rarely death. The risks of a DVT are highest in patients who are very obese, are on the contraceptive pill, who smoke and who have a long operation. One recent study of liposuction in nearly three hundred patients showed none of them suffered this complication, so fortunately it is rare. Overweight patients are also at a slightly increased risk of suffering from a chest infection after surgery.

A more common but less severe complication of liposuction is that of contour deformity. The smooth skin contour is disrupted with the formation of an uneven surface. It is caused by too much fat being removed from one area adjacent to an area where not enough has been removed.

It occurs in only a small number of cases. Likewise, skin dimpling can occur if the suction cannula gets too close to the skin surface. If patients are not willing to accept this risk, they should not be having liposuction. There may also be some numbness in the skin of the treated area after surgery.

The scars produced by liposuction are very small, but they can sometimes become red, itchy and prominent for a while.

Some surgeons use ultrasound assisted liposuction. This is reported to have more effect on stubborn fat areas. It carries some additional risks. It can cause discoloration of the skin as it has a heating effect. It has even been reported to have caused internal damage to some deep structures as there is less tactile feedback for the surgeon. This is extremely rare.

LIPOSUCTION	
Cost	UK: £1,000 - £5,000 US: $2,000 - $10,000 (depends on areas treated)
Anaesthetic	General Anaesthetic
Hospital stay	1 - 2 days
Recovery	1 – 2 weeks
Risks	Wound infection Asymmetry Numbness Contour deformities Uneven skin texture and dimpling Abnormal skin pigmentation (uncommon) Damage to deeper structures Loose skin after large volumes of fat removal

15. Choosing a Cosmetic Surgeon

In the UK the NHS will fund some procedures, such as breast reductions for very large breasts. Financial constraints and increased rationing have significantly reduced the number of cosmetic procedures performed within the public system. Regional differences in availability also exist. Most people now have to pay for their own cosmetic surgery. In the UK there are a number of surgeons who offer cosmetic surgery privately. The best way to find a surgeon is to consult your GP. They will know the local surgeons, and should have some idea of what area they specialize in. It is much safer to find a surgeon this way than to look up ads in the yellow pages or on the internet. It is important not to be embarrassed about taking up GP's time for what some people may consider trivial. Their role is to look after your well-being, and this includes finding you a safe plastic surgeon for cosmetic procedures.

UK trained surgeons will have the initials FRCS or MRCS after their name. This means that they are a

Fellow or a Member of the Royal College of Surgeons. Surgeons who have completed a training course in plastic surgery and who have been examined by their peers on their practice of plastic and cosmetic surgery will have the initials FRCS(Plast) after their name.

In America a surgeon who is Board Certified in Plastic Surgery has similarly undergone an evaluation which includes an examination. This is designed to assess their knowledge, experience and skill in the specialty. Plastic surgeons who are certified by the American Board of Plastic Surgery and who are members of the American Society of Plastic Surgeons have undergone rigorous training and have been evaluated by their peers on their practice of plastic surgery, from both the technical and ethical perspectives

If you decide to have a cosmetic surgery procedure you should have at least one consultation with your surgeon in his outpatient clinic or office prior to the date of surgery. This is very important. It allows the surgeon time to examine you and decide if the surgery is appropriate. He or she will explain the operation to you, tell you what it involves, outline the benefits and warn you of the risks. They will explain how long the surgery will take, what type of anaesthetic is needed, and how long you will stay in hospital. They will give you some indication of the recovery period. This whole process may take about half an hour of clinic time. Most surgeons will give you time to think over what you have been told and then review you in clinic after a few weeks. This process is very important, and all good surgeons will make time to ensure you fully understand the whole procedure.

Sometimes a surgeon will refuse to perform the surgery you request. He or she may feel that the surgery is not appropriate for you. If this happens it is almost certainly done with your best interests in mind.

Glossary

Aesthetic surgery-

Aesthetic surgery is an alternative name for cosmetic surgery.

Abdominoplasty-

Alternative name for a tummy tuck.

Anatomical Implants-

Implants that are shaped like a tear drop. Also called shaped implants.

Areola-

The small circular area of coloured skin around the nipple.

Augmentation mammoplasty-

Alternative name for breast implant surgery.

Blepharoplasty-

Alternative name for surgery to remove the excess skin and fat from the eyelids.

BMI-

Body Mass Index. This is a ratio of a patient's weight when compared with their body surface area (estimated using the height). It is calculated using a chart of weight and height. A patient with a BMI of over 30 is considered obese. The risks of surgery are greatly increased when patients have a BMI of over 35.

Capsular contracture-

A fibrous capsule that forms around some breast implants. It changes the shape of the implant to a sphere. This can cause pain but often presents as a change in the shape of the breast. Surgeons have a grading system from one to four to measure the severity.

> Grade I: the breast is normally soft and looks natural.
>
> Grade II: the breast is a little firm but looks normal.
>
> Grade III: the breast is firm and looks abnormal.
>
> Grade IV: the breast is hard, painful, and looks abnormal.

The rate of capsular contracture can be reduced by using sub-muscular implants, using textured implants, using antibiotics and by minimal handling of the implants during surgery.

Deep Vein Thrombosis (DVT)-

This is a blood clot which forms in the deep veins of the leg. It is caused by prolonged periods of immobilisation, such as surgery and air travel. The clot can block the vein and cause painful leg swelling. This is treated with anti-coagulant drugs. Very rarely the blood clot can move from the leg onto the lungs via the blood stream. This is a dangerous condition called a Pulmonary Embolus (PE). This can cause severe shortness of breath and even death. The risk of a DVT is increased by obesity, smoking, the oral contraceptive pill, hormone replacement therapy, certain blood disorders and long surgery. The risk of DVT is reduced by heparin injections, wearing special stockings and using special foot or calf massaging devices.

Drain-

This is a small plastic tube which is left in the surgical wound. It allows any residual blood to drain out of the wound after surgery. This prevents a haematoma forming. Drains are usually removed the day after surgery. This is done on the ward by cutting any retaining suture and pulling gently. It is relatively painless.

Dressing-

A dressing is used to cover a wound after surgery. The aim of the dressing is to collect any discharge from the wound, prevent infection entering the wound, produce a good environment for wound healing and to improve the aesthetic appearance of the wound. Surgeons use a variety of dressings. Cotton gauze, paraffin coated gauze and modern polymer films are all popular.

Endoscope-

A small telescope fitted to a camera. It is used to look into body cavities and is often used for brow lift surgery.

Facial Nerve-

The nerve which supplies the muscles in the face. It emerges from behind the ear and spreads forward over the face. It is at risk of damage during facelift surgery.

FDA-

Food and Drug Administration agency. This agency regulates the use of devices such as breast implants in the USA.

General Anaesthetic-

This is a drug induced state of unconsciousness. An anaesthetist will use a combination of drugs and inhaled gases to put the patient into a state of sleep. When the patient is asleep they will control their breathing, level of consciousness, muscle tone and blood pressure. They will also administer analgesic drugs to reduce pain levels and amnesic drugs to reduce the patient's recollection of the procedure.

Haematoma -

A collection of blood that forms within a surgical wound. It is due to blood release from tiny vessels within the wound. It occurs after a small percentage of operations, usually within the first 48 hours after surgery. If the blood collection is not removed it can cause complications such as infection and skin necrosis. The wound is re-opened, the blood clot removed, and the wound is then re-sutured.

Hypersensitivity-

Abnormal sensation which can occur when the nerve to a tissue is damaged. It can occur in skin, ears, breasts and the nipple.

Hypertrophic scar-

A prominent scar. A small percentage of scars will become hypertrophic. They become red, raised and itchy. This often begins a few months after surgery. It commonly occurs in wounds on the chest and shoulders and in wounds under tension. It can be improved with the use of topical silicone, steroid injections, pressure dressings and massage.

Hyperpigmentation-

A darker area of skin due to an increase in the level of pigment in the skin.

Hypopigmentation-

A reduction in the level of skin pigment causing a pale area of skin.

Keloid scar-

A thickened, lumpy scar. This occurs in a small percentage of patients, often with dark skin or a predisposition that runs in the family. It is most common on ears, the chest and shoulders. It can be treated with steroid injections, silicone and pressure.

Local Anaesthetic-

Local anaesthetic is a substance which can be injected into a region of the body to block the nerves. This will eliminate the sensation of pain from this region of the body. The patient is still awake but will not feel any pain when a surgical incision is made.

Mammogram-

A breast x-ray to exclude breast cancer.

Mastopexy-

The operation to correct the shape of drooping breasts.

MHRA-

The Medicines and Healthcare products Regulatory Agency. An executive agency of the department of health in the UK. It regulates the use of breast implants in the UK.

Otoplasty-

Alternative name for prominent ear correction surgery.

Pulmonary Embolus (PE)-
This occurs when a blood clot, which forms in the leg, moves to the lung. This can cause shortness of breath and rarely death. It is a rare complication of prolonged surgery. The risk is increased by smoking, obesity, the oral contraceptive pill and some blood disorders. The risk is reduced by heparin injections, wearing special stockings and using special foot or calf massaging devices.

Ptosis-
Breast ptosis - another word for breast droop. Graded from one to three by surgeons, depending on the nipple position.

Eyelid ptosis – a drooping eyelid due to muscular imbalance.

Reduction mammoplasty-
Alternative name for breast reduction surgery.

Rhinoplasty-
Alternative name for the operation to improve the shape of the nose.

Rhytidectomy-

Alternative name for a facelift operation.

Seroma-

A seroma is a collection of lymphatic fluid within the surgical wound. Lymphatic fluid is essentially blood without the red cells. It is a viscous yellow fluid. It appears as a swelling around the wound within the first few weeks of surgery. It can often be removed by aspiration with a needle and syringe, though it can recur.

SMAS-

Sub-Muscular Aponeurotic System. A layer of tissue in the face which lies directly over the facial nerve. When pulled upwards during a facelift, it will lift the overlying fat and skin.

Subcutaneous tissue-

The layer of tissue directly beneath the skin. It consists of fat.

Textured implants-

The surface of most implants is made from solid silicone. Textured implants have a rough surface, with many tiny lumps on it. The rough surface is designed to prevent a capsule forming around the implant.

Umbilicus-
Another name for the belly button